Zero
DAYS IN SAFETY

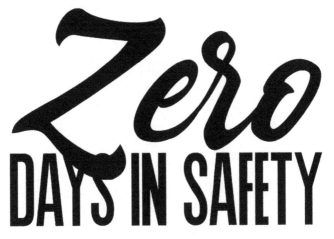

Zero

DAYS IN SAFETY

One Nurse's Journey into
Trauma and Recovery

David Foley, PhD, RN

Foreword by Mary Dolansky PhD, RN, FAAN

Zero Days in Safety
One Nurse's Journey into Trauma and Recovery

ISBN 978-1-7375813-0-7

Published by:
Frances Anne Publishing
USA

This book is dedicated to all students considering a
career in nursing.
You belong.
Let no one tell you otherwise.

For my mother and my father

ACKNOWLEDGEMENTS

I am so grateful for the opportunity to acknowledge a number of people who helped me create my life's narrative of safety. First, I thank my parents Ann and Ed Foley, who, so very long ago, worked very hard to provide their three children with the best life possible in our typical suburban enclave.

Next, I must thank my sister Ellen, closest in age of my siblings (the other sibling being my brother Ed). You watched over me as a small child and continued to do so on that fateful day of September 29, 2016. Ellen, Sister Dehlia was right. You would have made an excellent nurse. Much, much love and thanks to you.

I must also thank my favorite human Mr. Bill Pummill. Your selfless offer of help during my recovery meant the world to me. Although you know I would without question, I hope I never have to return the favor.

I also express my gratitude to my dear friend and colleague Sharon Wing. You are a nurse extraordinaire who has made an enormous impact on my teaching/nursing practices. You will forever be immortalized as "Our Lady of Perpetual Pain Relief."

Sincerest thanks to Chairperson Dr. Vida Lock and the other members of my dissertation committee. I can never repay your kindness but assure you I will work diligently to pay it forward many times over to future students.

I also thank the amazing Dr. Mary Dolansky from Case Western Reserve University's Frances Payne Bolton School of Nursing. I appreciate your vast knowledge and caring, unselfish desire to mentor others so very much.

I next acknowledge the contributions of the teachers at William Foster Elementary School and throughout the Garfield Heights School System. Thanks to your collective efforts, I felt more than ready to move on to college and face the world.

I also thank Dr. Pamela Combs, who inspired me to further my nursing education. Through many instances of Divine providence, our paths continue to cross, and will hopefully do so many times in the future.

Thanks in turn to my dear friend—and former boss—Betty Hickle. You are a true maven and the pureness of your unconditional love for others is nothing less than inspiring.

Much gratitude to the wonderful Reverend Charles and Mrs. Mary Jo More and fellow parishioners Ralph and Judy Bates for often being, at least in my mind, true examples of Faith and God's love in action. How grateful I am to each of you.

Lastly, I thank God for his watchful care over me in all things—especially on the afternoon of September 29, 2016. So many things could have gone wrong, but didn't, thanks to His guiding hand so I could move forward...in safety.

CONTENTS

Contents

FOREWORD

STORYTELLING IS A powerful pedagogical tool that enhances and sustains learning. David Foley's book Zero Days in Safety: One Nurse's Journey into Trauma and Recovery uses narrative storytelling to share the personal account of his journey into "safety" while at the same time teaching the core principles of quality. Readers of this book will gain an appreciation for many facets of healthcare, including the often difficult transitions patients experience, the importance of therapeutic communication, and the complexity of the healthcare system.

With a creative twist, the book also highlights dimensions of the profession of nursing and the unique contributions of nursing to healthcare. Specifically, the experiential narrative describes both the details of David's healthcare journey and presents his thoughts on injury, trauma, recovery, acute pain, anxiety, despair, and depression. The unfolding of the events of David's life, defined by the nexus of his core value of safety and alignment of nursing philosophy, is an innovative way to teach and inspire the next generation of nurses. The story provides a cleaver interlacing of the philosophy of nursing, nursing theory, and the experience of men in nursing that provides students an appreciation for the uniqueness of the profession. Experienced nurses, as well as nursing students, will undoubtedly enjoy reading this narrative.

Along with safety, the other QSEN competencies (Cronenwett et al., 2007) of patient-centered care, evidence-based practice, quality improvement, teamwork and collaboration, and informatics come alive within the context of David's patient-care experience. Nurse educators can use the book as a teaching modality to help students link QSEN competencies to better patient outcomes. They can also use the book to teach nursing philosophy and highlight the often difficult to teach "soft" skills of therapeutic communication, empathy, and relationship building. Using the book and providing time for reflection and innovative thinking, faculty will bring a refreshing approach for students to envision a new era in healthcare.

Kudos to Dr. Foley for sharing his life journey in "safety" to inspire undergraduate and graduate nursing students to appreciate quality and safety competencies and engage in the attainment of the Quadruple Aim: to enhance the patient experience, improve population health, reduce costs, and improve the work-life of health care providers, including clinicians and staff. Enjoy the story and the learning!

Mary A. Dolansky, PhD, RN, FAAN

Sarah Cole Hirsh Professorship
Associate Professor & Director of the QSEN Institute,
Frances Payne Bolton School of Nursing
Associate Professor, School of Medicine
Case Western Reserve University
VA Quality Scholars Program (VAQS) National Advisor
Senior VAQS Faculty VA Northeast Ohio Health System

Cronenwett L, Sherwood G, Barnsteiner J, et al. (2007). Quality and safety education for nurses. *Nursing Outlook, 55(3)*, 122-31.

Sikka R., Morath J.M., Leape, L. (2015). The quadruple aim: care, health, cost and meaning in work *BMJ Quality & Safety, 24,* 608–610.

ABOUT THIS BOOK

THIS TEXT IS intended to be read from several complimentary perspectives. Written in narrative form, it can simply be viewed as the story of a trauma patient who suffered a potentially life-threatening injury and the ensuing journey to recovery. From that broad viewpoint, the general public can vicariously experience the realities of interfacing with our complex, often frustrating, and constantly evolving healthcare system. Within that framework of hyper-turbulence, the reader may relate from a strictly experiential or reflective point of view. In other words, they may recall times when they experienced extraordinary care, encountered a 'difficult' healthcare provider, felt excluded during conversations among interdisciplinary team members, or simply felt like a number floating through a system.

From a different perspective, the story can be read by Nurses—or Nurses in training—who nobly provide care to patients across the continuum of care. They may read the account of physical and psychosocial injury with interest, especially as the context shifts from a Nurse living in a safe, insulated suburban existence to brokenness in a large urban hospital's Level I Trauma Center, then tracing the experience to the inpatient unit, home, outpatient surgery center, outpatient therapy, and follow-up office visits. The sheer number of those transitions will hopefully capture the exhaustive, yet rewarding, nature of recovery.

Despite the opportunities to improve healthcare pointed out in the narrative, an optimistic theme is woven throughout the story: the privilege of seeing former nursing students in practice. What Nurse educator wouldn't delight in the opportunity to see their students in action, albeit without the context of personal injury? Nurse educators celebrate with their students during time-honored Pinning and Graduation Ceremonies, but other than impersonal contact through social media, they seldom cross paths afterward. Still, this narrative acknowledges the contributions of Nurses and Nurse Educators everywhere—a powerful team who practice, educate, research, lead, and advocate.

As presented, I had the chance to receive direct bedside care from many current and former students and see the training they received in the classroom, nursing skills lab, and clinical rotations come to life. As I lay nearly helpless, watching these current and former students integrate classroom knowledge with technical skill was a unique and fulfilling experience, but one I hope no one would envy. Nonetheless, seeing former students in action affirmed my mission to continue my work in nursing education from a deeper, richer perspective.

This book is thus also intended as an educational tool to enhance general public knowledge and encourage students and faculty to look beyond de rigueur standards of nursing education. In doing so, they may push much deeper to explore the affective domain, celebrate nursing theory, test the waters of cultural competence, and begin actively to construct their professional nursing identities. I vividly recall the many times students smiled with delight when they completed their first blood pressure and other more complex medical skill checks but watched with concern as they struggled to see the value of developing the more nebulous and seemingly complex skills of therapeutic communication and psychosocial assessment. Perhaps this story will encourage students, Nurse Educators, and Nurses in practice to focus, even if just a bit, on less concrete, psychomotor-based skills and deeper into the 'art' of nursing, if nothing else to promote the highest standard of safe patient-centered care possible.

I hope the reader will consider the importance of safety in their own homes and healthcare settings. However, from the broadest perspective, I share my own narrative of safety, a concept that since childhood provided a sense of structure, comfort, and security that ultimately defined me. That strong focus on safety eventually became a cornerstone of my nursing and administrative practices.

In part to cope with the sudden and traumatic externalization of my locus of control, I discuss the many times I drew upon my Faith, family, and other sources of support, including the power of nursing theory. In particular, my nurse theorist hero Dr. Betty Neuman has been a source of ongoing inspiration. I had the opportunity to speak with her during my graduate course in Nursing Theory, where she freely and generously shared her theoretical perspective with my classmates and me. Despite painful injuries and the prospect of a long, protracted recovery, the Neuman Systems Model helped me organize my thinking and make plans to access all available resources and, in doing so, affirmed my desire to continue to affirm Nursing Theory's great utility with students at all levels.

This book is thus not intended to be a textbook but rather an experiential narrative that presents my thoughts on injury, trauma, recovery, acute pain, anxiety, despair, and depression. Information about the QSEN Competencies, nursing theory, and Erikson's Stages of Psychosocial Development is mentioned within the context I recalled them in my compromised state. My recall, thoughts, and feelings have not been sanitized in the interest of scholarly writing.

From a purely educational perspective, perhaps the most compelling opportunity when reading this text is to reflect on the Quality and Safety Education for Nurses (QSEN) competencies of Safety, Patient-Centered Care,

Teamwork/Collaboration, Informatics, Teamwork and Collaboration, and Quality Improvement. In my opinion, internalization of these competencies should be a cultural imperative in nursing education and practice, as according to the QSEN website: www.QSEN.org,

> The Quality and Safety Education for Nurses (QSEN) project addresses the challenge of preparing Nurses with the knowledge, skills, and attitudes (KSAs) necessary to continuously improve the quality and safety of the healthcare systems within which they work. This website is a central repository of information on the core QSEN competencies, KSAs, teaching strategies, and faculty development resources designed to best support this goal. (Reprinted with permission from the QSEN website www.QSEN.org).

Although I previously could not articulate them in such a fluent and organized manner, utilizing these competencies had already been an integral part of my administrative, nursing, and teaching practices for nearly three decades. When I discovered the QSEN Institute's website, I felt like I had found a comfortable home, and I 'moved in' immediately. I am now grateful for the chance to share my thoughts with you.

Lastly, this text highlights a man's foray into the world of nursing. Entering into the profession as a former hospital administrator in my early 30's, my career in nursing has often felt like an intrusive sojourn into someone else's world rather than a fulfilling career path. Nevertheless, I was inspired to become a Nurse based on the kind and compassionate caring I observed by the many Nurses in the areas I supervised. Their rich demonstrations of the art and science of nursing strengthened my perspective as an essentialist whose philosophy was rooted in compliance, fiscal responsibility, and, most importantly, safety. I am so thankful each day that so many nursing colleagues and students have chipped away at that shield of pragmatism to allow me to create my own nursing narrative as one who cares deeply and passionately about the students and patients I serve.

Onward….

Dr. David Foley, Summer 2021

PROLOGUE

A S A VERY small child in late 1969, I remember how happy I felt each day when my father arrived home from work. Such child-like joyful exuberance is something many of us rarely experience as adults, but for young children, it seems effortless and unstoppable. He worked quite a distance from our home, and in those pre-cell phone days, traffic and weather made his nightly entrance a bit unpredictable; nonetheless, hearing the dull thud of his car door was a highly anticipated daily event in my small world. I scrambled to the kitchen door to greet him, as his arrival meant our small family was now complete.

While he changed clothes, my mom moved into high gear to corral three children away from our Zenith black-and-white television and to the dinner table. Frenzied activity followed as we settled into a warm, structured routine that included dinner, conversation, homework, a story or game, more TV, and despite many objections, bedtime. Life during that wonderfully structured pre-school existence meant fearlessly living only for the moment, with no awareness of danger and no care for the concerns of tomorrow.

Our home, a small bungalow in a typical post-war suburban enclave, was my entire world—safe, secure, and seemingly untouchable. Nothing bad happened there. As I grew older, I came to understand my father's arrival meant he was returning from work, where he earned money to provide our food, shelter, and in essence, our security. Mom managed the home front while dad ventured out into the unknown each day. That division of labor and responsibilities perfectly met the needs of our small family.

As a curious Kindergarten student two years later, I noticed my dad wore a vinyl pocket protector emblazoned with his company's name. I was immensely proud I could read it, and come to think of it, my parents were quite proud I could read it too. They encouraged their children to read anything and everything, which fueled my desire to devour all knowledge in my path. My older sister, who shared my passion for learning, aspired to be an elementary school teacher and taught me many skills beyond my level of development, something that my teachers quickly noticed.

One day, I asked my father if I could take his pocket protector to 'Show and Tell' to inform the other students in my Kindergarten class where he worked and teach them to read the name too. He politely declined, stating it contained too much important information, but after much begging, took it out of his pocket and showed it to me. Its many contents included a small screwdriver, magnet, and index cards containing many words written in his precise, draftsman-style printing. One word perched atop several of the cards, caught my attention: safety: S-A-F-E-T-Y. After a few failed attempts, I said "safety!" and then asked what it meant. He studied me for a moment and then carefully explained it meant doing things so no one would be injured at work.

"You mean like falling down and getting hurt?" I asked quite seriously. "Yes," he replied, "like falling down and getting hurt." I was immediately horrified, as I had fallen down and skinned my knee on the pavement, and it *really hurt*. Worse yet, a little boy up the street fell and had to go to a terrifying place known as the hospital to get *stitches*. Did that happen to people where he worked? I hoped not, as I would never want that to happen to anyone, let alone him. I felt relieved as he went on to say he was on a safety team that tried to keep people from 'falling down and getting hurt.' They did this by teaching employees how to properly clean their work areas and do their jobs in the safest manner possible. He said our family should also make sure our home was safe and asked if I was interested in helping him. Of course I was, so he drafted me on the spot and we talked about how to make our home a comfortable, safe place to live. He made it seem so exciting and important, of course I wanted to help!

I couldn't wait to tell my class all about safety at the next 'Show and Tell.' Despite my enthusiasm, my dad still wouldn't let me take his pocket protector to school. Yet, he took out a clean index card and wrote down some of the words we had discussed: his company's name, safety, environment, accident, education, and team. I took the card to school and was very proud to stand in front of the class to share with pride how my dad was making his—our—world a safer place.

My teacher was impressed and told each of us that it was our responsibility to promote safety in our homes and classrooms. While the whole class listened intently, she talked about fire drills and how important it was to remain calm, get in line, and follow the leader in the event of any emergency. She even discussed specific things we could do to make our classroom environment safer. In our young minds, this novel concept of safety seemed so highly intriguing.

As the years progressed, I understood how much promoting safety at his workplace meant to my father. However, not until I was in college did I fully realize his involvement began around 1971 when President Nixon created the Occupational Safety and Health Administration per executive order. Perhaps my father's personal focus on safety was in part a reaction to a wave of a renewed national focus on safe working conditions. I can't be sure, but I know performing job duties safely was essential to him. Often the line between work and home became blurred as he told our family stories about on-the-job adventures—and misadventures.

We eventually discovered he was a member—and ultimately team leader—of his company's safety team that conducted formal environmental rounds and promoted safety education. Safety campaigns quickly became cultural imperatives within the company, so much so that they advertised the number of accident-free days (and thus the number of days in safety) on bulletin boards within the building. At the end of each accident-free day, the total number of 'Days in Safety' increased. Whenever an accident occurred, the number was reset to zero, and the bulletin board displayed the ominous message 'Zero Days in Safety.' My dad shared that, thanks to efforts to educate and promote awareness, many times the number of days in safety reached 50, 60, 100, 200 or more, but then an accident would occur and the number would return to zero, free to begin its hopeful ascent at the conclusion of each subsequent accident-free day.

The company encouraged all employees to carefully monitor workplace conditions, suggest areas for improvement, and participate in debriefings in the unfortunate event an accident occurred. Despite his optimism, my father sometimes expressed disdain for employees who declined to participate in any safety measures.

Regardless of the cause, whenever an accident happened at work, he arrived home with a particular look on his face. It wasn't just a typical look of a tired thirty-something man who had labored hard all day to feed his family and was simply glad to be home. It was instead a look of anxious concern and the result of an incredibly stressful day. Sometimes his expression conveyed the leftovers of a disagreement with his boss, but more often it meant someone had gotten hurt, and that they hadn't simply 'fallen down and skinned their knee.' Someone's father, son, or husband was the reason the bulletin boards declared 'Zero Days in Safety.' His look conveyed that a serious accident could have—or did—result in a serious, potentially life-threatening injury that meant loss of income, lifestyle, and on one terrible occasion, near loss of life. Such serious injuries absolutely horrified me—but from a safe distance. I knew I was safe in my home, far away from danger. In our little world, bad things simply didn't happen, or at least not to *us*.

As the years passed, I watched as each family member, whether they liked it or not, was drafted onto my father's safety team. He became irritated when my mother jerked a plug from the electrical socket, reminded us to keep our rooms clean and clutter-free, expressed disdain at the 'toxic fumes' emitted by my sister's nail polish remover, and was so disappointed when my older brother got into an accident with our beautiful blue Buick Skylark. Standing in the driveway, he listened intently as my brother earnestly recounted the cause of the accident. Although my mom backed my brother's story completely, my dad simply stood and stared at the smashed right rear fender for an uncomfortably long time. Without saying a word, he stoically turned and walked away with the same look on his face when an accident occurred at work. That was a terrible day, and for the record, the damage was not my brother's fault. How dare someone hit our car and intrude into our well-insulated and safe existence! It was one of those rare occasions during my childhood that our home's bulletin board read 'Zero Days in Safety,' and I simply couldn't believe it.

As I moved into adolescence and early adulthood in the early-mid 1980s, my father and I argued about many things, but often about his myopic focus on safety. By that time, my young mind no longer viewed the concept through wide-eyed wonder; it was now an annoyance. I just wanted to be young, carefree, and enjoy my expanding world that now included school, church, friends, and eventually my first job.

When he advised me to drive carefully and make wise decisions, I often roared back, "why worry so much? You seem obsessed! Safety is important, but so is *living*. You can't manage everything." Delightful banter with his 5-year-old son begging to look at the cards in his pocket protector eventually morphed into a middle-aged man scolding his adult child. "Use your head…what were you *thinking*?" he often said whenever a potential breach of safety was observed. Such chiding really irritated me. "Come on…*loosen up!*" I told him.

What had I done to deserve such critique anyway? Most of the adults in my childhood and adolescence called me one of the 'good kids,' as validated by good grades, solid attendance, and even a few awards. I certainly did my part to maintain a respectable existence in our stalwartly safe world. I did my homework, attended church, and kept curfew, each day returning to the warm safety of our home. My father's concerns were about things that *could* happen, but that was for someone else—not *here*. Nevertheless, 'near misses' like the time I *almost* got into a car accident did happen, and I saw the same look he gave my older brother as he walked away, stoically shaking his head.

To be honest, those were terrible days too.

Despite our spirited debates, I somehow survived childhood, adolescence, and most of my adult life without a serious accident. My own billboard screamed 'Thousands of Days in Safety!!!!!' and I worked to create my adult world bounded by a safe and secure home front. Nevertheless, I still returned to the safety and comfort of my childhood home often, hoping I had made my parents proud with each career milestone.

"Safety is a top priority," I told my employees in the 1990s, but upon reflection, those words seemed a bit hollow. Even though I was acting in the role of supervisor or classroom leader, I knew many employees and students did not share my passion for safety. They only wanted to *feel* safe and know *someone* was out there doing the work to ensure they were. Nonetheless, I initiated a similar 'Days in Safety' campaign, and some employees thought it was great. A simple glance at the 'Days in Safety' total was all they needed to know. If the number was high, things were going well, and they were safe. "An 'idiot light' for safety," as one of my older employees put it.

Occasionally accidents did happen at my workplace, serving up a worrying wake-up call. Now facing 'Zero Days in Safety,' my employees could also no longer celebrate the passage of another workday without injury or malfunction. They were reminded that just glancing at the 'Days in Safety' bulletin board might not be enough. Instead, they needed to monitor their work areas more carefully and report any potential breaches in safety immediately to prevent a reoccurrence.

Emphasizing safety at the hospital or within a patient's daily nursing care plan was fine for the workplace or academic setting, but I gave little thought to such matters on my home front. Why should I? I lived a life with minimal risks. My concept of safety permeated my psyche to create a false sense of security that defined my carefully constructed existence. Bad things *did not happen*, not in my world.

All of that changed, however, in one moment on a beautiful autumn afternoon in 2016. On that day, the last vestiges of childhood naiveté were swept away by a very brief lapse in judgment as I attempted a rather mundane home improvement project. In the moments after an unexpected and potentially life-threatening fall from an extension ladder, I was enveloped in a feeling of amazement. Even though I sat up dazed and with searing pain, I asked myself a deceptively simple question: *what had just happened?* There was no need to ask, however, because I already knew the answer. I didn't know the specifics yet, but something terrible had happened. I was no longer safe. But wait a minute…something like this couldn't happen to me….could it? After a few moments of reckoning, I quickly came to embrace the fact that it certainly had, and I was in serious trouble.

In disbelief, I realized my own billboard now read 'Zero Days in Safety!!!' When my father learned the news, his face would have that familiar pained look, but this time not about a co-worker but me. How could I face *any* of my family, friends, employees, and students who heard me decry so often that "safety is a top priority"? Thoughts like *"you should have done a simple safety assessment before you started…" or "you should have known better than work alone. It's better to work in pairs!"* raced through my mind. *"You fool! Why didn't you follow your own advice?"*

Was I a hypocrite? I hoped not.

As I dealt with the trauma, unspeakable pain, and long recovery, it took every ounce of my faith in God, education, experience, and support of family, friends, co-workers, and students to come to terms with what happened. A bad thing had happened to me, and they all knew it. My sense of security would never quite feel the same, but the healing power of time helped me create a new narrative, albeit within a different and more pragmatic worldview. After surgery and many months of occupational therapy and emotional recovery, I celebrated the addition of each new day on my personal safety billboard.

Zero days in safety, one day in safety, two days in safety, three days in safety…

Zero
DAYS IN SAFETY

PART I

THOUSANDS OF DAYS IN SAFETY

CHAPTER 1

PARASITIC OVERAGE

"...the best way out is always through."
Robert Frost

S TARTING WITH MY first successful 'Show and Tell' experience, I was hooked. I loved being in front of the class and often wonder why I didn't pursue an undergraduate degree in education. I think somewhere along the way I heard a strong, unified message: teaching didn't pay enough and there just weren't enough jobs in our area. "If you want to earn a real living, don't be a teacher....you'll never find a job!" I recall a trusted adult figure saying.

Nevertheless, continued exposure to my father's successful safety education campaigns, excellent Sunday school teachers, and the caring devotion I received from many public school teachers instilled a love for learning that eventually grew into a passion for educating others. It took me several years to initially unearth my calling, but I have now been blessed to engage in the unique, symbiotic process known as teaching for over 18 years. The process is bi-directional and ever so rewarding; I learn just as much from my students as they do from me. The work is hard, but each time I leave the classroom, I feel uplifted and ready for the next step in my journey of personal and professional growth.

My frame of reference wasn't always so optimistic, however. Before entering the teaching profession, my child-like sense of inquiry was nearly obliterated by the day-to-day drudgery of working as a hospital administrator. From 1995-2000 I leveraged the career potential of earning a Master's degree in Public Administration to quickly work my way up the ranks at a local publicly-funded hospital, ultimately chasing my tail as Director of Operations for a large business unit. Like my father's existence years before, the events of each day set the tone when I returned home. If things went well, I arrived carefree and relaxed. Days marked by an adverse patient outcome, poor financial news, or employee misadventure meant a quick dinner followed by a march to the computer for follow-up emails. Luckily, I worked with a group of incredible people, and more often than not, we were able to do damage control and move on with our evening.

Occasionally something quite adverse happened that could not be so quickly resolved. Such deleterious events required a 'root cause analysis,' or a highly deliberate and very laborious attempt to determine a negative outcome's true source. Sometimes we performed these analyses for a batch of improperly billed patient accounts, an act of misfeasance during a medication administration, or even the events leading to an unintended patient death. In any case, the process of determining the cause of the breach in safety usually boiled down to human error. Effective policies were in place, and adequate resources had been provided to support a safe workplace, so employees choosing workarounds or, worse yet, blatantly ignoring safe standards of practice were more than likely the reason. "What were they thinking?" I often echoed my dad's words as I coalesced with the rest of the team to determine the most appropriate course of corrective action.

I self-imposed a 'total accountability with no excuses' standard to model sensible and safe workplace practices. If the boss wasn't willing to be a role model, how could the employees be expected to do so? Although I drew the line at overtly advertising safety by wearing a pocket projector like my father, those with whom I worked knew safety and 'coloring within the lines' were extraordinarily important to me.

My big break came in 1997 when I was promoted to an administrative position supervising the highest volume group of clinics in the hospital system. My self-imposed standard of safety was quickly tested just one month into this new position, as word swept like brushfire throughout the hospital of the unexpected arrival of The Joint Commission (TJC). I knew TJC was a vital body that sets standards of practice in hospitals and published its annual list of National Patient Safety Goals (NPSG). Those goals were usually developed in response to clusters of negative occurrences in health care settings across the country and were highly relevant to daily clinical practice and administrative operations.

A colleague quickly educated me that TJC had arrived for an unannounced accreditation visit and was there to assess our compliance with their standards. She told me the surveyors would undoubtedly ask me and others on my staff to provide evidence that we had made reasonable, good faith efforts to meet the NPSG and other expected standards of care. *"Oh great," I thought, "I've only been on the job three weeks but have to face the music for the previous administrator's work."* I felt enormously unprepared and toxically stressed.

Luckily several highly seasoned Managers and Coordinators in my operations were well familiar with compliance surveys. They sprang into action, and everything went fine. After TJC surveyors left, one of my Coordinators looked at me wistfully and said, "so much of what we showed them was window dressing. Wouldn't it be nice if we actually *did* everything we presented to the surveyors every day?" In making that one statement, she unknowingly provided me with the central theme for much of my future administrative practice. We (especially me) already knew safety should be the linchpin of any respected healthcare workplace. Why shouldn't we weave safety into all aspects of our daily work and, in doing so, hitch our wagon to a rapidly burgeoning phenomenon known as creating a 'culture of safety?'

In future meetings, we recognized that a solid foundation was already in place, even if only from a reactive perspective. Before any TJC inspection or review, we were advised to proactively report all adverse outcomes that fell within the reporting period. Doing so seemed to convey a sense of openness and organizational transparency. Following any such untoward event, it was expected that a robust administrative response ensued to determine the cause(s) and put effective controls in place to minimize any chances of a reoccurrence.

Some of those happenings were classified as 'sentinel events,' or highly distressing occurrences resulting in serious injury, a decline in bodily/mental function, or worse yet, loss of life. I began any investigation by seeking input from the nursing staff, whom I grew to respect as the collective glue that held our operations together. I quickly learned if I wanted to get the real story, *ask a Nurse.* Their knowledge, expertise, caring, compassion, and focus on safe, patient-centered were deeply inspiring.

As we dug deeper, I realized my prior graduate studies in health care administration prepared me well for my administrative responsibilities. Still, it didn't take me long to realize how little I knew about adopting a proactive approach to creating a culture of safety within the clinical setting. Several Nursing Coordinators and Directors, collectively responsible for our operations, helped me fill in the hazy, gray area between administration and safe patient care. "I don't think that policy will work, and here's why…" one of them told me. "Please don't cut that position from the budget; it will really hurt our clinic flow…." another said. "We don't like that piece of equipment. It might be the best price, but it won't work for us," yet another pleaded. After a few early missteps, I took their advice, and our clinic operations became the 'go to' destination for Nurses seeking a supportive environment where everyone's opinion mattered. Members of the interdisciplinary team were indeed talking, collaborating, and proudly creating a *culture of safety*.

Several months later, I was summoned to the Senior Administrative Board Room for a mysterious meeting with the hospital's Chief Operations Officer (COO) and Chief Financial Officer (CFO). My initial sense of intrigue was squelched when the COO apologized that he had to "lower the boom" about our budget. In the middle of his passably civil discourse, the CFO interrupted and blurted out that my clinical operations were "…in the red thanks to all your nursing staff who are nothing more than ***parasitic overage*** to your budget. I know they take care of people, but they don't bring in any money, and you have way too many of them!" His words bounced across the vast, magnificently polished wood conference table and made me angry. I recoiled, found my voice, and fired back with as much sincerity and alacrity my 32-year-old experience and perspective would allow. I was unceremoniously silenced by the

COO, who of course, agreed with his senior colleague. "Now go back and trim your budget! Get rid of some of the dead weight!" was his charge, and with a virtual pat on my head, the meeting ended abruptly.

I fled to the cafeteria and was surprised to find several of my administrative peers licking their wounds over coffee. They had already had their meetings with the COO/CFO duo of flatulence and received the same message. We offered each other words of sympathy and agreed to stick together. Although we were all bound by the common administrative purpose of fiscal responsibility, we were also unified in the respect we held for our Nurses and commitment to quality, safe patient care.

Curiously, by the next day, this shocking and unexpected assault on my nursing staff no longer made me angry but instead stirred a sense of intellectual curiosity I hadn't felt since college. Although our CFO was right in that Nurses circa 1996 had few opportunities to provide billable services, they *cared* for our patients/customers/consumers and seemed to know so much about what was needed to make the system work better. Their labors were so noble; they certainly *had* to be more than a drain on the bottom line.

Over the next week, my curiosity grew into a frenzy. I just had to know more about what made Nurses tick, so I spoke with—and even shadowed—many of my nursing staff. Still, I wanted to know even more, so seated in my office one non-descript afternoon a month later, I decided to become a Nurse. Just like that. I had no idea what it took to become a Nurse; I just knew I wanted to be one. My plan, rooted in nothing less than sheer naiveté, quickly took shape: work as an administrator by day and pursue nursing studies during evenings and weekends. Oozing with self-confidence, I was sure I could do it and was quickly accepted into one of our area's last remaining hospital-based evening-weekend programs.

As suspected, the years 1997-2000 were nothing less than glorious insanity. Nervously eyeing the clock during a 3 pm meeting and then running to the car to race across town to attend class or clinicals. Every day I prayed no one would notice my life's descent into chaos and compensated by going into work an hour early to remain abreast of my work responsibilities.

Who needed sleep anyway?

I have no idea how, but I successfully kept my new adventure a complete secret, even from my closest friends and family. I was incredibly proud that despite the odds, I was also able to remain incognito at work. My co-workers and senior administration had no idea I was enrolled in nursing school until two months before graduation when an administrative co-worker visiting a clinical site saw me in my student uniform and cheerfully spread the word to as many employees as he could by Monday morning.

During that period of clandestine intellectual exploration, I often dashed breathlessly into the school to start an evening class or clinical rotation with absolutely no time to spare. On more than one occasion, I even changed into my student nursing uniform in my car. To add to the stress, from the outset, my instructors, seemed to question my motives for entering the profession. "You already have a good job," one of them asked me, "why are you here?"

"I admire Nurses and just decided I wanted to become one," was all I could reply. I knew about budgets, compliance, and human resources but desired to see these standards from a nursing perspective. As my coursework continued, staffing shortages no longer meant open positions on a spreadsheet. They meant toxic stress for overworked Nurses and, worse yet, potentially unsafe care practices. A break in the supply chain was not only a performance improvement opportunity; it was a potential breach in accepted standards of patient care.

These lessons reshaped my administrative perspective in so many ways. During working hours, I spent more and more time with Nurses and less with my administrative peer group. 'Managing by walking around' is what one of my old textbooks called it. "Tell me about your job," I would ask someone, and with some gentle Socratic questioning, gradually shifted the conversation to the challenges of providing safe, quality patient care within fiscal restraints. Perhaps sensing my sincerity, they opened up to me, and I never felt any of them were complaining; they just wanted to serve our patients to the best of their abilities. As my training continued, I understood that nurses could provide valuable input into staffing levels, customer service initiatives, and even equipment choices. Since they had so much contact with our patients, it made sense they should be empowered to speak up and perform their duties as autonomously—and safely—as possible.

I'm not sure when I decided to leave hospital administration behind, but I think it was sometime in the spring
of 2000 as word of my foray into nursing had spread
throughout the organization. The senior officer who
made the 'parasitic overage' comment began to avoid
me intently. I can only speculate on his thinking, but
his silence seemed to communicate I was a defector who
no longer belonged in administration. It was the first of
many career experiences where my gender, education, or
administrative experiences seemed to place me at odds
in the nursing workplace.

Strangely I *did* feel like a bit of a traitor within my
circle of administrative colleagues. I almost felt like someone who had been eavesdropping, heard way too much,
and was now at risk for taking insider secrets to the other
side. The decision was mine as to which team would hold
my membership, and in the end, the choice was simple.
I felt incredibly energized as the profession of nursing
beckoned me. I felt empowered by a new perspective and
sensed my education and budding clinical experience
would take me on quite an adventure.

On graduation day, I was one of only a handful of
men who claimed their coveted nursing pin. As I processed down the aisle, my parents looked at me with
loving pride. A few steps later, my gaze shifted to the
female faculty member who had asked me, "what are you
doing here?" but this time my thoughts silently roared
back, *"I am here to claim my nursing pin like all the others,
nothing more and nothing less. Now, will you please stop
being so elitist? All I want is to enjoy this day with friends*

and family like the rest of the students!" Finding my seat, I recall thinking that nursing instructor might be just as exclusionary as the COO and CFO at the hospital, but from a very different perspective. *"None of you scare me anymore. Maybe you never did,"* and with that silent proclamation, I relaxed and enjoyed the rest of the ceremony and ensuing festivities.

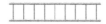

During my three-year nursing program, there were so many points when I wondered if the stress of feeling ostracized by some of my instructors and the fatigue associated with fifteen-hour days was worth it. About a week after graduation, some Nurses at my workplace answered that question when they hosted a congratulatory potluck luncheon for me. Although I had never been invited into their inner sanctum, requests for meetings were nothing new. I had walked past their lounge many times as laughter—and delicious aromas—wafted into the hallway. They shared a unique bond and never seemed to pass up an opportunity to gather in celebration. On this day, a trusted staff Nurse asked me to step into the lounge to address some concerns the Nurses were having, and I unblinking complied. As the door opened, I was stunned into complete silence by a loud "SURPRISE" followed by many rounds of "congratulations!" all from a large group of dedicated Nurse professionals.

In response to shouts of "speech…speech!" I could only manage to give a few words of thanks for the inspiration they provided me to begin my journey into nursing. Their acts of caring, leadership, advocacy, and courage had deeply touched me. I told them their work was so crucial to the mission of the hospital (*"and no…. you're not 'parasitic overage' to the hospital's budget"*).

I concluded my brief comments by asking the rhetorical question, "does this mean I'm one of you now?" "Well, sit down and let's see. Can you handle this?" they replied and handed me the first of many prized gifts—a plastic bedpan emblazoned with each of their signatures. "Be sure to find a way to put it to good use!" someone called out, and we all laughed heartily. That gathering was such an incredibly meaningful event, one I enjoyed far more than the school's pinning ceremony. I was about to become one of *them,* and their kind validation made the stress of the previous three years suddenly seem like just a bad memory.

As I scanned their faces, I realized I was looking at a distinguished group that included licensed practical, registered, and advanced practice Nurses who had provided care for thousands of patients, delivered babies, fought for prescriptive authority, and in general, worked each day to make healthcare safer and more effective. I admired them and wanted to walk in their footsteps.

"What's next, the Vice President of Nursing?" someone called out, and everyone laughed again. *"No,"* I thought. *"I only want to be a Nurse, but my own kind of Nurse."* Safety, firmly embedded in my psyche since childhood, was now poised to become an integral part of my nursing practice. I looked forward to finding ways to provide top-quality nursing care that was cost-effective, efficient, informative, yet most importantly, safe. I aspired that no Root Cause Analysis Team would ever have to investigate a sentinel event that resulted from my actions.

Only time would tell, but days in safety continued.

Incidentally... I still have that bedpan and count it among my prized possessions.

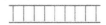

I took the 'nursing state boards' only one month after graduation in June 2000. One of my classmates called me a few days before the test and said she scheduled a week's vacation so she could completely relax after taking her 'boards.' *"Oh, to have such a luxury,"* I thought. The day's events leading up to my exam perfectly embodied the chaos of nursing school. I made my testing appointment for 12:30 pm and slipped out of the office for an "off-site meeting." I drove across town to a standardized testing site and took the exam in one hour on an ancient computer with a monochrome screen. After seventy-five questions, the computer screen went blank, and the hard drive began to whir. Relief washed over me, as according to my soon-to-be colleagues, that usually meant a passing score had been achieved. The printer spit out a single sheet of paper, and I nervously examined it. It contained no information and was quickly whisked from my hand by the test monitor, who told me my test results would be mailed to my home within a month. I jumped in my car, grabbed lunch from a drive-through, and managed to slip back into my office for a 3 pm meeting. *"A week's vacation, huh?"* How long could I keep up this break-neck pace?

My nursing students often lament about waiting 24 hours for expedited nursing state board results. In those days before electronic notification, the nearly month-long wait for 'snail mail' communication seemed interminable. I nervously checked my home's mailbox each day and, on a beautiful June summer's evening about a month later, found an envelope with "Board of Nursing" listed as the return address in my home's mailbox. I ripped it open and stopped after reading the letter's salutation: *We are pleased to inform you...*

Though dusk was heralding the end of another long day and several of my neighbors were visible, I whooped and danced in the middle of the tree lawn, my mind racing with hope, optimism, and possibilities. My administrative position just hadn't felt like the right fit for quite some time, and in reading that one sentence, I felt a sense of total relief and a right-sizing of my universe. I decided right then I would leave hospital administration behind. That night I mulled over the idea of keeping my administrative position and exploring nursing as a second, part-time evening/weekend job, but then summarily dismissed the plan. The document I held in my hand was the ticket to a life of new adventures, and I decided it was best to move on.

I knew there would be challenges in starting over again. Still, nothing could possibly be as stressful as being held responsible—and often feeling solely accountable—for the actions of several hundred employees. My various administrative positions had required me to do so for several years, and I was just tired of it.

I soberly reflected, however, that *my* nursing actions could now be the source of a serious error, and someone might receive a call about *me*. Instead of managing budgets, tackling human resource issues, and leading hospital safety rounds, I would soon be a Nurse at the bedside, a front-liner who must ensure safe patient care. What could possibly be more exhausting yet fulfilling? I felt I just had to take some time to explore nursing, especially since I never wanted to be known as one of those teachers or administrative Nurses who 'never touched a patient.' I decided I needed to enter the nursing workforce to gain experience and perspective, so when I spoke with other Nurses, I could relate on a meaningful and collegial level.

A few days later, I drew in a deep breath, opted for a complete life reboot, and resigned. My legs felt so heavy as I walked down the hallway to my boss's office, but I felt free once I told her. My boss Betty, however, was genuinely shocked. We had worked so well together, handling many employee issues, surviving budget cuts, and passing TJC reviews with flying colors. Many people stopped by my office to offer well-wishes, but to also ask the same question: "why….?" "You're so good at what you do. Why would you want to leave this?" Betty said she would hold my resignation for two days to give me the chance to think it over, but I told her there was no need—I was leaving and, to the shock and amazement of everyone, left my administrative position for a full-time career in nursing.

When I left previous jobs, I focused on making sure that budgetary and personnel issues were in good order, and this time was no exception. However, I now benefited from three years of nursing education that provided me with insight into the importance of cultivating and maintaining meaningful human relationships. As a result, an integral part of my exit strategy this round was to give attention to the people around me, making sure my relationships with them were in good order. I shook hands, tried to resolve hard feelings, and even asked many of them for advice. Their words of wisdom were highly valued, as I was starting from ground zero in the role of novice Nurse and needed every drop of knowledge I could get. I knew the transition from administrator to Nurse would not be easy, but their words came back to me as a powerful source of encouragement over the ensuing months.

On my last day in October 2000, I expressed my total admiration to the Nurses in my department, once again reminding them they "were the glue who held it all together." Despite the hugs and well-wishes, turning off the light in my office for the last time was difficult, and the ride home seemed very lonely. Nevertheless, I continued to quietly celebrate my decision to venture out into a different world. Nursing ushered in a new era, but not one of ease and comfort. I would work harder than I ever had before, entangled in a new form of stress that was so demanding yet somehow satisfyingly comforting.

I saw things from a very distinctive perspective from the moment I entered full-time nursing practice. I joined the profession in 2000, the height of a severe nursing shortage, so wages were extraordinarily high with employment opportunities everywhere. Nevertheless, even during chaotic shifts when I worked without a break due to short staffing or was mandated to work overtime, I realized I had no desire to return to my administrator role. Against the advice of colleagues who encouraged me to take a permanent hospital-based nursing job, I instead took a position with a temporary staffing firm. Although they usually only hired more seasoned Nurses, the recruiter carefully perused my administrative experience and convinced a local hospital to offer me a 12-week temporary contract.

On my very first day on the job, a well-meaning beleaguered nursing supervisor approached me and said something like, "we are critically short-staffed….would you mind taking a patient assignment today? I will check in on you from time to time, and I *promise* we will start your orientation very soon."

I never saw her again.

I took the whole patient assignment and muddled my way through that first shift. I did not commit any errors, but that was because I had the insight to realize I was consciously incompetent in many areas and, as a result, asked many questions. My previous experience serving on critical incident or root cause analysis task forces taught me one of the primary reasons for serious patient errors was staff members' reluctance to ask for help. In those early days, I asked for help…*frequently*.

It didn't matter if any of the other Nurses talked behind my back or looked down on me for proceeding with careful deliberation. I was there to provide competent, *safe* patient care. The safety billboard at my dad's work emerged as a symbol for frequent reflection. True to his mission decades earlier, I vowed I would not be the one to commit a severe error and be responsible for our unit's billboard blaring 'Zero Days in Safety.' I knew taking an assignment as a new graduate without an adequate orientation was not ideal. Yet, I proceeded with caution and somehow made it through that assignment—and many more over the next two years—without committing any serious errors.

I forged ahead, tapping into my administrative skills to create what many referred to as my 'interesting' approach to nursing. I strove to be an organized and efficient Nurse who read policies, called pharmacy for advice, and volunteered for safety rounds. My confidence grew, but I still carefully double and triple-checked procedures, especially those with which I lacked adequate experience. Only after many, many rounds of self-checks did I allow myself to transition into conscious competence on a skill. After all, I had read Patricia Benner's fascinating book *From Novice to Expert,* which in part conveyed it may take up to seven years to progress from novice to expert. So I restrained myself from feeling too confident. I had a long way to go, and I knew it but moved carefully ahead.

Days in safety continued...

CHAPTER 2

COMMITMENT PHOBIA

*"It is the danger which is least expected that soon-
est comes to us. It is the flash which appears, the
thunder bolt will follow. It is the misfortune of
worthy people that they are cowards."*
Voltaire

AFTER WORKING AS an agency nomad from
2000-2003, I took a full-time job as a Registered
Nurse at a local government facility. I was initially
reluctant to do so because working for the temporary service was the perfect antidote to my commitment phobia.
To my surprise, I had enjoyed the freedom of working
on a contract basis, especially after being tied down in

administrative roles for so long. The agency viewed me as a dependable Nurse with a solid track record, so if I wasn't particularly enamored with my current assignment, I knew they would allow me to move on to the next one with no questions asked. Some of this moving on was involuntary, as certain assignments had a 'residency rule' that essentially allowed temporary staff to work there only for a defined period and then face the decision to either join their team or leave. Those were times when exiting required a good deal of contemplation; on other occasions, egregiously unsafe care practices made me flee without hesitation. As I pushed my way through one particularly harrowing shift, I began to wonder if being an agency Nurse was such a wise decision after all.

The kerfuffle occurred one warm spring day when Katie, a very polite Nursing Assistant (NA) who was graduating from her RN pre-licensure program in just six weeks, approached me red-faced and breathless. "Have you seen Jess?" she almost shouted as she stared at me with glistening, pleading eyes. "No, I haven't," I replied. *"It's a very small unit. She should be here somewhere,"* I thought. "Maybe she stepped off the floor for a minute," I said and smiled reassuringly at Katie but thought ruefully, *"with only two RNs on duty, she should have told me she was leaving the floor."*

"Well, until she gets back, will you please help me with a few things? I have everything else covered, but I'm not sure about the settings on the IV pump in Room 4, and I need someone to double-check my insulin..." she said. I quickly interrupted, "OK, wait, why are *you* worried about the IV settings in Room 4 and asking me to double-check insulin. I know you're graduating soon, but you're still a NA, and you shouldn't be doing those things here…"

Katie burst out crying and sobbed, "I wish I would never have agreed to this. I want to go HOME!" Staring open-mouthed and incredulous, I asked her to sit down at the Nurses Station. "Katie, tell me what's going on. I'm sorry you are upset, but I think you should tell me.…"

"It's Jess! She said she had somewhere to go and gave me fifty dollars to cover her patients. She's been so good about letting me do things so I can practice my skills. I've hung lots of IVs for her and passed a ton of meds. She was here though when I did those things, and now she's not, and I'm *scared!! What am I going to do???*"

Oh dear.

"Katie, is Jess in the hospital? Let's wait for her to get back. As soon as she gets here, we'll sort all this out…"

"No, she's not in the hospital!!! She went to a wedding and said she wouldn't be back for a few hours. She told me to cover for her! She has a pager but told me not to use it unless it was a real emergency!"

"A few hours? A real emergency? Well, I'm sorry we're going to have to bother her royal incompetentness, but I think this is a real emergency!" "Well, Katie, I think this falls under the category of 'emergency.' I'm not going to take responsibility for all the patients on this unit. It's just not a safe practice, and besides, I haven't received nursing report on any of Jess' patients. Page her and let her know…the secret is out."

Jess returned the page a few minutes later, and after a quick update from Katie and a return flow of hot, steaming profanity, Jess declared she could not possibly be back for at least two hours, and we should 'be cool' and cover for her. I tried to take the phone to speak with Jess, but she abruptly hung up, leaving a very pale and motionless Katie. "I'm going home NOW!" Katie practically screamed as she began to weep.

"Katie, I'm calling the Nursing Supervisor. I think Candi is on duty, and she's pretty understanding. I'm sure she'll help us figure this whole thing out. It's just not safe for me to handle all these patients myself. I'll overhead page her. Why don't you go into the Break Room and relax for a few minutes?" Candi returned my page almost immediately, and I did my best to explain the situation as parsimoniously and diplomatically as possible. She listened silently, said "I'll be right there," and materialized almost instantly.

Feeling far freer to talk in person, I took Candi aside to recount the situation in as much detail as possible. "She went to a wedding???" she asked and wearily leaned against the wall. "Just when I thought I had heard everything..."

"Yes, Candi, amen to that. I have seen a lot in my career, but nothing like this!"

"Candi, we have some really sick people up here, and I just can't take all this on by myself. Can we get a float until Jess returns?"

"UNTIL SHE RETURNS???" Candi interrupted, almost shouting. "She's outta here...I'll send someone over to help from the ICU as soon as I can. In the meantime, where's Katie? I wanna talk to her!"

"Candi, she's just a college student who was led down the wrong path," I soothed. "I know you have to probably report her, but I think she's had enough for tonight."

"David, just go back to work and let me take it from here, ok?" Candi said very directly.

"Yes ma'am! With pleasure!"

I threw myself into caring for my patients, silently praying for the end of this horrendous shift to come quickly. About an hour later, I saw a metallic flash disappear around the corner and sensed trouble. I glanced down the hall just in time to see Jess, wearing a cocktail dress, dash into the Staff Lounge. She presented almost immediately to the Nurses Station wearing scrubs but in full hair and makeup. "What's your problem, dude?" she snarled. "You need to get a life, and just remember… snitches get *stitches!*"

Yes. She really said that. I had heard of the expression, but no one had said it to me before, and to be honest, I was very concerned. Jess was one tough customer, and I suspect it was a role she had played well throughout her life.

She charged down the hall and rudely attempted to dismiss the ICU Nurse, who by now had passed medications and, with Katie's help, had each of the patients settled in for the night. Despite Jess's pleadings and thinly-veiled threats, the ICU Nurse (I wish I could recall her name) didn't leave but stood her ground and called the Nursing Supervisor. I'm not sure what Candi said, but the ICU Nurse beckoned Jess to the phone, and after listening with stone-faced intensity, Jess hung up and said she was "outta here." She quickly collected her things and, on her way, out the door, landed a parting shot at me, seething, "I'll see you soon...I PROMISE! I needed this job!"

At the end of the shift, I gave the oncoming Nurse report and then requested Security escort me to my car in the interest of my safety. I wasn't the least bit concerned about perceptions, even when the Security Guard snickered just a bit when he realized I was the Nurse who called. On the long, silent drive home, my thoughts raced, and I asked myself one question over and over...*had I done the right thing?*

After a fitful night's sleep, I continued to feel very secure in my decision, a conviction that grew steadily over time. From a clinical or administrative perspective, a Nurse abandoning their assignment and asking a Nursing Assistant to 'cover' duties obviously outside their scope of practice was in clear violation of our state's Nurse Practice Act. There was simply no 'looking the other way.' Safe patient care must always prevail, and I knew that.

I thankfully never heard from Jess. I heard she took an out-of-state travel nursing assignment, but I hoped she was just not seeking a geographical cure; instead, I hope she took some time to reflect on her actions and made some badly needed changes. I never knew what happened to Katie, but I assumed she graduated and entered into nursing practice.

I called the agency and let them know I couldn't go back to that site again. In addition to this capstone nightmarish incident, I had been asked to take assignments of 10-12 high acuity patients in recent weeks, and I decided working there was simply too risky. Based on my work ethic and excellent attendance record, no questions were asked, and I was welcomed at the next similarly understaffed facility with open arms. I soon decided, though, that enough was enough, and it was time to settle down. I applied for many nursing opportunities but ultimately decided to accept a full-time, permanent staff Nurse position at the local government agency.

The decision raised many eyebrows within my circle of friends and former work associates. During my first two years in the profession, many of them never lost an opportunity to inquire if nursing was what I really what to do long-term. Some even predicted that once I "got it out of my system," I would return to a career in hospital administration. In their eyes, that seemed to be the most logical career path, especially since I could tap into my rapidly expanding cache of clinical knowledge to add richness and depth to my administrative expertise. For now, however, I sensibly took the full-time nursing position, primarily due to the minuscule 5-minute commute and excellent fringe benefits.

Not surprisingly, I quickly adapted to the disciplined routine of government work, as such order was nothing new to me. After only five months as a staff Nurse, our Quality Assurance Nurse, a resolute woman who hardly spoke to *anyone*, pulled me aside and whispered that the previous month I had entered the most chart notes of any Nurse in a three-building radius. Curious, she took the time to look at several of my chart entries and informed me she was impressed with both the quality and quantity.

Wow.

She went on to say I had been 'drafted' onto the Quality Improvement/Safety Committee and asked if I had any experience with Root Cause Analyses. "*More than you know,*" I thought but simply told her, "Yes, I have." She said the committee looked at errors mainly from the perspective of workflows and policies and that they "…tried to keep personalities and politics out of the mix." Although reticent at first, I thoroughly enjoyed the committee's meetings and, unable to help myself, volunteered to format summary reports that were well-received by senior administration.

A few months later, I found myself being summoned to the Director of Nursing's office. She said she had been "keeping her eye on me" and encouraged me to apply for a Nurse Manager position on a unit with an extremely high level of patient acuity. She was very persuasive and told me she was looking forward to "seeing what I could do" with the unit, especially given my background in leadership and administration. "I pulled your resume from your personnel file and was so pleased with what I saw. You'll do just fine!"

Although I was flattered with the recognition, my heart sank, as I knew my life would change if I took the position. As opposed to bedside nursing, the role of Nurse Manager carried the responsibility of passing numerous inspections: mock inspections by The Joint Commission (TJC), consultative TJC inspections, *actual* TJC inspections, the hospital's Environment of Care Rounds, and my personal favorite, the hospital's Patient Safety Rounds (PSR).

Not surprisingly, safety was a common thread that wove its way through these reviews and the entire medical center's culture. As a Federal agency, the level of scrutiny was far more intense than at my previous hospital. Although I usually felt energized by such challenges, it felt quite unnerving to live under the myopic scrutiny of wave after wave of inspectors. Despite our best efforts to prepare, it was humbling when they found 'deficiencies,' and I was expected to submit an effective action plan to achieve immediate compliance and prevent reoccurrence.

As they were simply the most intense, most Nurse Managers especially balked at the very mention of PSR, finding them to be labor-intensive, embarrassing, and inconvenient. In short, PSR required us to work until late in the evening while an interdisciplinary inspection team assessed every nook and cranny of our unit for cleanliness, compliance to policies and procedures, and of course, any potential breaches of safety. I liked PSR and, in unspoken opposition to my colleagues, not only tolerated these inspections but welcomed them. My staff and I worked very hard to meet accepted standards, and it showed. When a deficiency was noted, I thanked the inspection team and indicated my interest to return to a state of compliance as quickly as possible. I didn't resist but instead welcomed the critique and acknowledged the opportunity to collaborate on rapid-cycle performance improvement.

Growing up in our household's culture of safety was partially responsible for any initial success in my foray into nursing management. I also gained much insight from the courses in my Masters of Science in Nursing (MSN) program. More than anything, the MSN curriculum called for me to lean into, not shy away from, critique, and I grew even more interested in compliance, performance improvement, and education.

I strongly felt the healthiest way to promote a culture of both safety and quality was to be resilient and open to feedback, and that strategy served me well. After three successful years, my unit was often cited as an exemplar of a "culturally transformed workplace," with low staff turnover, high patient satisfaction scores, and many days in safety.

I certainly didn't achieve this recognition alone. Simply by word-of-mouth, our unit attracted the best and brightest Nurses in the facility, and together we made an outstanding team. We frequently referenced our collective efforts at maintaining a state of "rolling preparedness" for TJC, PSR, and other inspections, meaning we were ready to be inspected anytime. Once the TJC *did* show up for an unannounced visit, and our advanced preparation paid off. We were calm, fearless but most importantly... ready.

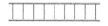

My unit was also a popular destination for Nurse Educators, who brought groups of pre-licensure nursing students from local schools to complete a required clinical rotation. I enjoyed working with the instructors to orient the students to our unit and pair them with Nurses who were genuinely interested in educating others. Based on positive feedback from the students, one of the clinical instructors approached me with a life-changing opportunity: would I consider taking a clinical group myself or teaching an introductory course in the nursing resource lab at their local community college?

I took the plunge and taught what I thought would be just one course. Standing in front of the class in the Nursing Skills Lab on my first day, I found myself tapping into the sense of child-like, untainted exuberance during my first grade 'SAFETY Show and Tell' topic. The nursing students matched my enthusiasm, and I realized I had unexpectedly found my life's calling. I favored educating through 'storytelling,' and my students seemed to respond to that style of pedagogy. I presented the required content but did my best to place it within the context of real-life examples, and they loved it. That initial experience as a Nurse Educator impacted me so profoundly that I soon desired to return to school myself. Exploring many options, I chose to obtain a PhD in Education with a concentration in Nursing Education.

After an initial inquiry with a local university, however, a unique employment opportunity arose within my current government agency, and the plan to continue my education would have to wait, at least for now. An ancillary site needed someone to move quickly into a senior administrative position, and I was encouraged to apply. During the interview process, my greatest challenge was to convince the selection committee, most of whom were male executive types, that I wasn't 'just a Nurse' but also had the administrative savvy to lead the hospital's most prominent business unit. In preparation for the interview, I compiled an extensive portfolio of letters of recommendation, transcripts, business plans, policies, and performance improvement exemplars.

As they hammered me with questions, I was transported back to my pre-nursing school days, where I sat at the large conference room table and struggled to defend my nursing staff from the omnipresent CFO/COO dynamic duo. Equipped with several years' of nursing experience, however, there was no hesitation in answering the interview panel's questions. After working as a full-time Nurse and Nurse Manager, I could do more than simply respond to questions about human resources, staffing, workflows, supply chains, policies, and quality improvement; I could emote to them from a much richer perspective. When they brought up understaffing and mandatory overtime, two critical issues the hospital was currently facing, I felt my response seemed authentic because I had experienced those same frustrations from the perspectives of a Nurse, Nurse Manager, and Administrator.

After several weeks of waiting, I forgot about the interview. I knew the wheels of Human Resources turned very slowly in government agencies, and I frankly assumed they had gone with another candidate. One day out of the blue, my phone rang, and the Human Resources Specialist informed me I had been selected. I happily accepted, realizing any personal academic endeavors would have to wait—at least for now—so I could pursue this challenge.

I refused to give up teaching, however and continued as a part-time evening/weekend faculty member at a local school of nursing. I was unsure if I'd have the energy to continue my newfound 'hobby,' but feedback from students and other faculty pushed me to keep going. I found teaching to be a wonderfully fulfilling experience. The nursing faculty were now *colleagues,* and we shared stories from the expanding suitcase of our collective experiences. The commonality of our classroom experiences resulted in collegial banter similar to the chatter I'd heard in the Nurse's break room several years earlier Now I was a small part of that, and it felt so right.

Just as I had with the clinical expertise of my nursing co-workers, I highly respected the collective knowledge of the nursing faculty. Many faculty had—or were pursuing—doctorates, and it didn't take long for the education bug to bite me again. After just two successful years in my administrative role, I decided it was time to return to school to pursue doctoral studies in nursing education. Despite a flawless TJC review, new program developments, and several human resource victories, I realized this administrative position had run its course and that furthering my education was clearly the next destination on my horizon.

As those who have pursued doctoral degrees know, the doctoral program would be an all-consuming, labor-intensive, multi-year journey. Although I aspired to be Dr. David Foley, I was well into my 40's when I began, and I started the program with a mixture of self-doubt and regret. I languished in an uncomfortable space, rapidly cycling between two reoccurring narratives of self-doubt: "why hadn't I done this earlier...if I had started when I was 35, I would have been done by now!" and "can I do this?" I also wondered if the inner circle of nursing faculty would indeed welcome me as a full-time faculty member. Throwing all caution and doubt aside, I applied.

During my admissions interview, I faced a panel of distinguished interdisciplinary faculty who attempted to determine if I was suitable for doctoral studies. Two of the panel's members were from the School of Nursing, and they took turns asking me questions about my philosophy of education. After an hour, I sensed the interview was waning, and one of them asked me the final question: "In just a few words, why do you want to pursue doctoral studies, David?"

"My answer is two-fold. I want to sharpen my critical thinking and see what I can do to help educate diverse groups of nursing students."

"Well, I think you're just a short step away from achieving both goals," she said as she stood, shook my hand, and winked simultaneously. Knowing that 'short step' would take several years, I accepted her affirmation in good faith and went home to plan. Would it be possible for me to go the distance, let alone enjoy this journey, even just a bit?

Time would tell.

CHAPTER 3

HOME AT LAST

The world owes you nothing. It was here first.
Mark Twain

EARNING A PHD would require careful planning and a significant lifestyle change, so I sold my large home and drastically reduced my spending habits. Since I had no desire to incur any student loan debt, I accepted a full-time 'lecturer (lowest in the academic ranks)' position to take advantage of the staff development (i.e., free tuition) benefit. Despite the anticipated emotional and financial speed bumps associated with transitioning from administrator to doctoral student, I sensed the risk was certainly worth it.

From the outset, I found existing in the dual roles of teacher and student to be a dynamic, interactive process that resulted in a period of joyfully chaotic personal and professional growth. However, stress was more often eustress in this new life, not the toxic distress caused by budget meetings, personnel issues, or patient complaints. Although I knew I would work hard, I could simply leave it all behind and go home when I left the university at the end of the day.

To make matters even more interesting, I started the doctoral program and my new position as College Lecturer on the same day. During that first semester, I worked two 16 hour days each week. At 5:30 am on the first day, I parked my car near the School of Nursing building and immediately felt my personal sense of safety threatened. I felt highly uneasy during the dark, lonely walk from the parking garage to the bus stop over 1,000 feet away, but when I reached the safety of the brightly lit station, my worries ceased. *"Why worry?"* I thought, and within weeks quickly incorporated the large urban campus into my narrative of safety. I doubted anything bad happened there either, *especially* in the shadows of the Nursing Building.

Days in safety continued.

Two days a week, I rode the shuttle bus to a nearby hospital to teach students in the clinical setting, only to return to the School of Nursing quite exhausted at 4:00 pm. I changed out of my uniform, answered emails, had a very quick meal, and then stepped across the hall into the classroom as a doctoral student. Luckily, the School of Nursing shared the same building with the College of Education, so I reveled in the luxury of the micro, 100-foot commute to school. I felt for the other students in my cohort who traveled to work each morning and had to fight rush hour traffic to attend evening classes. Their perseverance was inspiring.

Knee deep in the second month, I began to doubt if I could manage the long hours for one semester, let alone three years. My internal dialogue battled back and forth between *"did the person responsible for making out the teaching assignments do this on purpose?"* and the more positive and pragmatic *"at least the tuition is free."*

I mentioned the distress of that exhausting first semester to the School of Nursing's administration years later and heard a chorus of "why didn't you say something? We would have changed your schedule!"

Really…

I was enculturated into nursing during the waning days of the 'nursing instructors eat their young' era and emerged with enough awareness to know it was best not to make waves. Instead, I chose to hunker down, brace for impact, and persevere. As College Lecturers were the lowest class on the academic food chain, I sensed it was best to simply stay out of the way of senior faculty and administration. They were a distinguished group that seemed to have tastes, style, and habits that were all their own, a common currency of the profession only they truly understood. Thanks to being around so many Nurses over the years, I *sort of* understood my academic colleagues, but only heavily filtered through my own lens. I resolved to finish the program, learn as much as I could, and become one of them. Only then could I possibly help reshape the culture of nursing education, even if just a bit.

I knew this would be an intensely productive time in my life, and there was no room for complaining. Thankfully family and friends were incredibly supportive, and their words of encouragement seemed to make the stress a bit more tolerable.

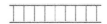

The doctoral journey was exciting and effervescent but filled with many obstacles, the most obvious of which was the omniscient, omnipresent, and omnipotent leviathan known as my dissertation. The best advice anyone gave me was to pick a dissertation topic I truly loved since, by the time I finished, I would certainly not only hate it, but thoroughly *despise* it. I took their advice and resolved to search for a meaningful topic through a very deliberate, intense process of introspection about my personal, subjective views of nursing education.

As time went on, I reflected that my students didn't observe the delineations of 'senior vs. junior' or 'academic vs. clinical' faculty. In their eyes, we were one unit. To them, we were simply faculty, the 'them' who possessed the common currency of clinical experiences and advanced degrees they desired to obtain. Despite my perceptions of the different classifications of faculty, to the students, I was simply part of 'them,' and the students were resolved to survive our program and enter into nursing practice. Such emerging revelations about social strata in nursing academia set the stage for my doctoral research.

I thus logically chose the concept of 'social capital' as my dissertation's organizing framework. In essence, I discovered that similar to my entry into the nursing profession, each of my students brought their own varying degrees of such capital (especially their previous educational experiences heavily influenced by culture, economics, and other factors) in tow as they started nursing school. As I moved forward with the dissertation process, I very practically chose to explore various factors that added to—or detracted from—passing the NCLEX-RN (the nursing state board examination) on the first attempt.

I knew researching this topic would help me reconcile my own nursing school experiences by proposing meaningful curricular enhancements to help nursing students who were male, of color, or those with limited English proficiency (LEP). As a member of one of those groups, I felt an incredible sense of purpose as I conducted my research.

Settle the score, so to speak.

I recalled the instructor calling me out on my first day of nursing school, saying, "you know, others may be happy about more men in nursing, but I'm not. Why are you here? Not too long ago, it wasn't like this…" On that first day, I hadn't met any of my classmates but recall receiving sympathetic glances from the few who dared to do something other than stare unblinkingly ahead. Much younger and quite naive, I finally raised my hand and joked, "Well, would you like me to leave?" *See, you'll just have to win her over through humor,* I thought, but my smile quickly faded.

My instructor's face clouded, and her eyes widened. "Don't give me any attitude, sir! I was only *joking!* What's wrong with you…can't you take a *joke?*" after which, I silently prayed the floor would open up and swallow me as the whale swallowed Jonah.

A few senior-level students were invited to speak with us first-year students, and they bore witness to the exchange. At the first break, two of them approached me saying, "don't pay any attention to her," reassuring me that she "meant well" and to "just give her a chance… she really is quite nice."

Nice? Compared to what, the latest health scare?

Thankfully, she and two of her colleagues were a self-contained epidemic within the faculty ranks. Like most Nurses, the faculty seemed overworked and a bit stressed, but nonetheless approachable. Most were quite supportive and seemed genuinely interested in treating all students fairly.

Note to self on my first day of orientation to the nursing program: study hard, graduate, and do something to make the field of nursing more welcoming to 'outsiders.'

But why did I feel like an outsider? My maternal grandmother's favorite saying, 'it takes all kinds of people to make a world,' inspired me to respect others, a sentiment that grew even as I advanced into adulthood and explored the world around me. However, my unfortunate impression on the first day of nursing school was that it took *very few* kinds of people to make up the world of nursing, and I wondered if I would survive until graduation, let alone have the staying power to make a difference. As a doctoral student, I actively tapped into these experiences and delved deeply into the concepts of social capital, social status, and in-group/out-group within the context of nursing education.

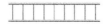

Flash forward, and here I was, a doctoral learner, exploring that 'note to self' on the first day of nursing school by conducting doctoral research on factors promoting—or detracting from— the success of diverse groups of nursing students. I was encouraged by some budding diversity in the classes I taught, but by and large, nursing appeared, at least to me, a profession still geared toward Caucasian females. I wished all of my students the best, but for those 'outsiders' who chose nursing as a career, would their individual and collective experiences be different from mine? I certainly hoped so.

I made a conscious attempt to explore the doctoral program's curriculum within the context of my own socio-cultural experiences. I found the readings—and subsequent research process—exciting and quite engaging. I looked forward to many deep dives into educational methods and the various factors that formed the social strata around me. I had already chosen the 'perfect' topic, the one I would love from the outset but might grow to hate by graduation. Yet as my research continued, I also thought it was essential to look at attrition rates, or the percentage of each of the three categories of 'non-traditional' nursing students (men, students of color, and those with LEP) who left the program before graduation.

Always the pragmatist, I recognized that since I was already comfortable with reviewing data, I would engage in quantitative research. I pursued a longitudinal, 5-year study on data collected within the School of Nursing where I taught, reviewing only de-identified information that painted an intricate composite of the students we served. As a local native, I became fascinated with the history and evolution of the surrounding school systems and was highly intrigued by the social and economic factors that shaped individual and community-based educational experiences. In doing so, I gained a much deeper appreciation from my 'podium perspective' that grew with every class I taught. I realized I was looking into the eyes of students from inner-city, inner and outer ring suburban schools systems, elite private schools, and for recent immigrants, schools from outside the United States. How could I make nursing school an engaging experience for all of them?

As soon as I gained knowledge in the doctoral classroom, I applied it to the nursing classroom. I learned techniques to 'flip the classroom' in yesterday's doctoral-level class and then 'hot off the presses,' used the same methods in the pre-licensure classes I taught the next day. As I gained knowledge about how adults learned, I strived to become a better teacher, both in the classroom, nursing skills lab, and clinical settings. After all, each of these three settings required—or should require—varied types of teaching methods. Better yet, each setting demanded culturally responsive teaching methods to avoid a 'once size fits all' approach to nursing education. Somehow I became known as one of the 'cool' teachers, one with whom you could speak openly and not worry about the conversation later. Was this really me? Was the 'do be' former high school nerd, hospital administrator, and tattered former nursing student finding acceptance and validation?

My love for teaching grew, and working each day was like finally trying on the perfect outfit. It just felt right. The students liking me was an added bonus and made coming to work an absolute pleasure. Although I rarely discussed my doctoral journey with my students, our unspoken comradery provided a collective understanding that fueled rich classroom discussion and a highly engaging, symbiotic learning process.

Back to reality! Comprehensive examinations and the Prospectus (i.e., the first three chapters of my dissertation) were on the horizon. Could I really *do* this?

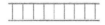

On a hot summer's night one month before the doctoral program began, I decided to assess my fitness for advanced studies through an impulsive decision to climb down a brambly steep hill behind my home. Who cares that I did very well on a standardized entry exam and aced the admissions interview! This *physical* challenge would determine if I had the resilience and stamina to complete the doctoral process. *Could I really do this?*

Although I enjoyed walking immensely, I had never really attempted hiking. Our family sometimes visited local parks for a 'hike' in the woods, but the visits were nothing more than walking on carefully maintained trails. Actual hiking meant a real challenge and a step into the unknown. I never really embraced sports in school or physical fitness as an adult, so I'm still uncertain why I equated hiking down a steep hill with the challenges of completing a dissertation. Still, in my sleepy suburban enclave, it seemed like the most challenging opportunity.

Throughout the hike on that stifling, hot July evening, I tripped, stumbled, and fell many times, including once when my foot slipped on a smooth rock, and I fell under the surface of the slimy green water. *"What was I thinking? Could I do this?"* I felt extraordinarily fulfilled when I reached the end, grappled up the bank, and found my feet planted firmly on the pavement. By car, the distance could be navigated in just a few minutes, but on that night, it took over an hour.

My evening walks were usually mundane and repetitive, with the same neighbors giving an obligatory wave and the same dogs barking their familiar tail-wagging friendly warnings. I would be hard-pressed to recall any significant detail on one of those walks, but today, I embarked on a new journey far from my well-beaten path.

During the wet, sloshy walk home, I ran into one of my neighbors who looked at me wide-eyed and asked, "What happened to you?" At first, I didn't understand why he asked the question but then followed his wide-eyed gaze from my damp, muddy shirt to my legs: streaks of blood ran from my knees to my ankles, and my shoes were caked with mud. Still enmeshed in abundant optimism at completing this self-imposed challenge, I hadn't noticed. My awareness restored, I shrugged off his concern and limped home, only then realizing one of the soles of my hiking boots was missing.

So that's why my foot hurt so much.

I quickly showered, applied a few band-aids, and then sat in a comfortable old chair in my garage while the sights and sounds of evening turned to dusk, then complete darkness. As I enjoyed that hot summer evening, I had no idea that just a few years later, I would lay severely injured due to a fall from a ladder just a few feet from where I was sitting. This time blood wasn't trickling down my legs from minor scrapes and bruises resulting from a hot summer night's misadventure, and the "what happened to you?" would not be resolved with a hot shower and a few band-aids, but several months of personal and professional trauma. With a sudden, traumatic thrust into the 'Patient' component of the 'Nurse-Patient' relationship, the promise held by my post-doctoral journey would be interrupted. I wouldn't be trying out innovations in the classroom, submitting a research application to the Institutional Review Board, or attempting my first post-doctoral publication.

Instead, I suddenly found myself quite suddenly residing at the bottom of Maslow's Hierarchy of Needs, first establishing I was alive, but then realizing with shock and disbelief I was unable to complete several of what the health professions call my activities of daily living: dressing, bathing, grooming, eating, and toileting. This was happening to *me?*

I discovered bad things did happen in my world.

Zero Days in Safety!

However, the silver living was immediately evident as I had personal care encounters with many current and former students, many of whom represented the evolving diversity I celebrated in nursing: those who were men, of color, and with limited English proficiency (LEP). They embodied *the very essence of my doctoral work,* and I was so joyful when they used their knowledge, skills, and ability to provide me with top-quality nursing care.

Despite my injuries, I couldn't help but revel in their success in passing the NCLEX-RN and accepting their first nursing job. The joyful realization that I had been just part of a team that prepared them to enter into practice quickly dissipated as I battled fear, depression, and an ongoing sense of panic over the traumatic externalization of my locus of control and sudden loss of independence.

My Faith in God and common sense told me I would recover, and my internal drive assured me I would do so sooner than the most optimistic estimates. Nevertheless, the journey was very hard. My recovery began even in the Trauma Bay when I heard so many assertions of "he's lucky...this could have been so much worse." As I lay there surrounded by so many people assessing my injuries, I felt very alone and yet, despite the unbearable pain, was thankful to be simply alive.

Over the years, I have constantly reminded my students of the importance of forging a positive Nurse-Patient relationship and that we must do our part to make that relationship succeed. I found myself, however, in a unique position. This time I was the Patient and many of the Nurses were my former students and alumni of various nursing programs offered by Nursing Schools and Colleges throughout our region and beyond.

They had all apparently learned very well, as their acts of caring and advocacy bolstered my strength and optimism. I later recognized I was also provided high-quality care by other members of the interdisciplinary team. Still, the pain and terror prevented me from embracing that realization until much later in my recovery.

Those next several months of my existence, firmly bounded by physical limitations and emotional pain associated with the sudden onset of a disability, gave me the invaluable opportunity to realign, and gather valuable perspective. In doing so, I become a better teacher and caregiver, and like my journey as a doctoral learner, the experiences were transformative.

Had I known what was to come, I may not have moved forward with my doctoral journal journey.

However, I celebrated an impulsive hiking adventure into the unknown on that night, and I relished my victory. It was an experience from which I would draw strength many times during my doctoral course of studies.

"Can I really do this...all of this?"

Yes, you can.

CHAPTER 4

LUCKY, OH SO LUCKY

To whom much is given, much will be required
Luke 12:48, KJV

THROUGHOUT THE FIRST few years of my teaching practice, I learned just how much I enjoyed interacting with beginning, first-semester nursing students. I eagerly explored many content areas with them including nursing theory, leadership, therapeutic communication, and caring. Other faculty balked at the challenge of teaching 'newbies,' after all, they really couldn't' *do* anything, but I highly valued the chance to witness milestone events like their first nursing physical assessment or coach them through challenges in an early Nurse-Patient relationship. These teachable moments provided many opportunities to shape their thinking from the inception of their nursing education; even more, I had the chance to help them begin to construct their nursing identities, a responsibility I did not take lightly. I continually referenced that 'note to self' from my first day in nursing school and vowed never to point to a student, even within the deepest recesses of my mind, and think—or worse yet say—"you don't belong here."

It has often been my observation that nursing students, especially during their first year, associate 'nursing' with performing what has been referred to one of my faculty colleagues as nursing's 'sexy' skills. To new nursing students, the profession is primarily defined by the dramatic and skills-laden scenes portrayed on many popular TV shows.

At this early stage in their education, I worked hard not to dampen their sense of wide-eyed excitement while exploring the nuances of the Nurse-Patient relationship, effective communication, or more complex concepts like advocacy or interdisciplinary collaboration.

In fact, during the first Nursing 101 lecture, I surrounded a mannequin, technically known as a low-fidelity patient simulator, by IV poles and several other types of medical equipment. As part of the teaching exercise, I removed each piece of equipment one at a time, telling the students what skill it is used for, continually reminding them that the patient, not the equipment, should be the focus of their nursing practice.

"Stethoscope…lung sounds are clear to auscultation anteriorly and posteriorly in all fields. An IV infusing D 5 ½ at 100cc an hour (they had no idea really what the meant, but I'm sure it sounded 'cool')." I dazzled them with jargon until the last piece of equipment was removed, leaving them face to face with just the mannequin-patient staring unblinkingly at them. I sat down in a chair placed near the patient's head and assumed its voice, making a simple, declarative command to the entire class: "help me."

Blank stares followed by an uncomfortably long pause.

Gently I continued, "Ok…there is a big YOU in parentheses. YOU help me. I'm speaking to all of YOU. Now what?" More uncomfortable silence, until one, maybe two, hands go up and ask to clarify the question. "Listen to the patient's request. *Please help me!* You will be asked far more complicated questions than this. Your patient is in distress and needs your help. How do you respond?" Another hand goes up, and a voice tentatively offers, "How can I help you, sir?"

With a sigh of relief, I validated their response and then launched into a discussion of Peplau's Stages of the Nurse-Patient relationship. With additional Socratic coaching, bit by bit, the students opened up and volunteered fuller and more empathic responses to the critical, open-ended request "help me."

By the end of the discussion, I acknowledged their aptitude for equipment and skills but asked them never to become task-oriented. I reminded them to look at the patient first, then the equipment. Even more, helping patients establish as much control over their illness as possible became a popular topic for discussion. "Please listen to your patients and empower them to make decisions in their own care" became one of my favorite sayings. I worked hard to refine this exercise over several years and later discovered many of the students recounted this experience as very impactful.

During the second year of their nursing program, I also had the privilege of teaching these same students Psychiatric-Mental Health Nursing. I thoroughly enjoyed facilitating the course, with its much deeper foray into the essential yet nebulous concepts of therapeutic communication and psychosocial assessment. Even more satisfying was assuming the role of psychiatric-mental health nursing clinical instructor, especially since I had the opportunity to work with the students in much smaller groups. The didactic and clinical courses were placed in the students' second year and thus yielded evidence of their growing confidence. My student advisees—and quite honestly many others—stopped by my office often to tell me about milestones in their nursing school experience, ranging from the joy of an unexpectedly positive clinical outcome to a tearful recounting of their first patient death. During these individual and small group discussions, I emphasized the need to approach patients with caring, even in the most desperate circumstances.

I was never sure how much these interactions impacted my students—if at all—until messages from newly-licensed student graduates trickled in through return visits, invitations to coffee, and social media postings. They continued to share their appreciation of the 'softer' side of nursing. The 'they' even included many of my male students who self-selected into the more 'technical' disciplines within the profession but seemed intent on sharing they were actually doing *nursing* and not just managing equipment. "Remember Professor Foley," one former male student who opted for a career in critical care began, "we have tasks to perform, but we must never become task-oriented. We are here to practice the art and science of nursing." He reminded me of how I often repeated my father's words back to him, but at least he was reciting the right message, and that made it quite satisfying.

I looked forward to finishing my PhD and leverage its strength to create an even more engaging classroom environment where students would feel empowered to explore. I also dreamed of impacting nursing curriculum as a whole, which I thought would be the most direct means to equip diverse groups of students to care for patients in the most culturally competent manner possible.

Such grand ideas.

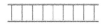

With a continued focus on my doctoral work, I pushed forward with a sense of passion and commitment I honestly didn't know was within me. I worked evenings and weekends and grew to call my office a second home. My family asked me why I just didn't come home, eat dinner, and then work on my dissertation there. After all, I had purchased a beautiful new computer for my home office but hardly used it other than answer emails and pay bills. I had no answer other than it seemed easier to pursue my studies at the university and then leave it all there. Once again, even if I arrived home at 10 pm each night, I was *home.*

My home front had always been an essential part of my existence and became the perfect solace for an introvert like me. A very public doctoral journey proved to be unbelievably exhausting, leaving little time to maintain my home's status as my private go-to place to recharge my emotional batteries. As the years progressed, it became even more critical to maintain the division between work-study and home. With stout resolution, the doctoral dominoes fell one by one: three comprehensive examinations, the prospectus defense, IRB approval, data collection and analysis, writing and revising, and finally, my defense. Write, re-write and repeat....so very often.

When the day of my doctoral defense finally arrived, I picked a small, intimate conference room that accommodated about a dozen guests. My dissertation chairperson advised me several times during the preceding months that she would not allow me to defend until I was genuinely ready; we would do all the hard work in advance. My defense was intended to celebrate my work and would be attended by my closest family, friends, and colleagues; failure in front of them was certainly not an option.

My immediate family asked me about a party. In my typical pragmatic fashion, I suggested a simple luncheon at the School of Nursing right after the defense so other family, colleagues, close friends, and students could join in the celebration.

On the chosen day, my guests were seated in the conference room while everyone else waited in a nearby classroom. When *the* moment arrived, the chairperson looked at me, nodded, and said, "Begin." This was my moment. I was surprisingly calm and made sure to make eye contact with everyone in the room. My sister, parents, my closest confidante Bill, and a few supportive colleagues were there. The experience was very emotional but rather fugue-like; I remember very little about that hour, other than I fought back tears when my parents and other guests were asked to leave the room so the committee could ask me questions. It prayed it would soon be over.

I acknowledged my committee members in a very grateful, dignified manner and prepared to offer what I hoped were logical, fluent responses to each of their questions. After a half-hour of spirited, good-natured grilling, the chairperson asked, "Does anyone have any more questions?" followed by a pause that seemed to last forever. "Ok, you may meet us in the classroom. Go wait there with your family and guests."

After a short wobbly walk down the hall, I entered the classroom, where the 50 people inside drew in a collective breath and applauded. *"Please,"* I thought, *"don't tempt fate…not just yet."* Their applause quickly abated when they saw I was alone, and we proceeded to wait for what seemed like a very long time for the committee to arrive. I couldn't look at any of them as they filed in. The chairperson, a fan of decorum, waited at least a full minute until the committee's presence silenced the room. "Ladies and gentlemen, it is my privilege to introduce to you for the first time *Dr. David Foley…*"

It was over.

I only heard one word of her remarks: privilege. The "Dr. David Foley" part of her statement was wonderful to hear, but I realized at that moment how lucky—and privileged—I was to have earned this credential and have my family present to share in such joy. Even then, however, the exuberance was tempered with an acute sense of responsibility to do something with my new credential. A verse of scripture came to mind "…for unto whomsoever much is given, of him shall much be required (Luke 12:48)." My heart was filled with gratitude, and I was ready to accept that Divinely-charged responsibility.

During the party, I looked around and felt like I was on the old TV show "This is Your Life." Promise and anticipation filled the air; life was looking up. With the help of family and close friends, we packed up the leftover food and went to my house, where the party continued late in the evening, ending only due to sheer exhaustion. The next day seemed surreal. Had I really defended? The house seemed eerily quiet, and I wondered…what now?

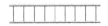

More joy, however, was close at hand as graduation day neared. I discovered I would be 'hooded' in the same spring commencement ceremony as my current students. When my name was called, the roar of my family, friends, and 200 students rising in unison and cheering is something I will count among my fondest memories. I recall the startled joyful, animated expression on my dissertation chairperson's face (a sedate, dignified administrator and scholar who actually *giggled*) and the quizzical look on the University President's face during the commotion. "Wow, he said! Who are *you*?" Although I served on one of his Presidential Committees, and he already knew who I was, I replied, "I'm Dr. Foley from the School of Nursing," and we both laughed. I think the ceremony's 'name reader' was just a bit flustered by having the proceedings momentarily interrupted, but she smiled and nodded approvingly as my extended moment concluded.

Lucky, oh so lucky.

I was visibly trembling as I walked off the stage down a long ramp, only then re-gaining a bit of self-conscious awareness that my hooding had just occurred in front of more than 5,000 people. The rest of senior university administration nodding in approval, and the School of Nursing's faculty, ever so dignified, sped by in a blur. In the distance, I saw my students, many of whom were still on their feet clapping and cheering.

As I made the final turn down the last aisle toward my seat, I looked up at my family high in the stands, right in the spot they claimed by arriving an hour early so that they could have the best view. My mom couldn't stop waving, and my dad, usually more stoic, waved and smiled himself. Following the ceremony, my family took me out to the restaurant of my choice, the same place we patronized the night of my high school commencement 30 years earlier. There was something so comforting being in that familiar place with my family, celebrating another graduation, only this time in a more mature state. So many familiar places had disappeared in the past 30 years, but this restaurant was still there to offer its silent acknowledgment of my achievement. Life could not get any better. I was filled with gratitude and looked forward to a return to rampant normalcy.

But then...

CHAPTER 5

THE POST DOC CRASH

**The forecast was cloudy with extended periods
of consciousness, followed by a stitch in my side
and a sense of impending doom swelling to a sym-
phony of demolition...**
Edward Morris

OTHER RECENT DOCTORAL graduates warned
me about the "postdoc crash," something they
described as an ominous, vacant feeling of "now
that I've graduated, where do I go from here?" At first,
being addressed as "Dr. Foley" was a tremendous psychological shot in the arm that overcame any sense of
foreboding. Still, as I was assured many times by senior

nursing faculty, it didn't last long. They were right. The post-doc crash *would* happen, but how soon?

Weeknights without classes and life without the dominating presence of the dissertation process seemed dull and boring. What impacted me most, however, were the long, vacant weekends. For approximately three years, I spent nearly every one of them at my downtown office, where I found I could get so much more done in such a distraction-reduced environment. I hadn't realized it, but the solace had become strangely addictive.

Now there was no one around but my cats and the first entire post-graduation weekend unveiled a previously unnoted evolution in my personality and disposition. Before my doctoral journey, I enjoyed staying home, watching TV, working around the house, and just giving myself time to rejuvenate after the workweek. My post-doc weekends now seemed eerily quiet and interminably long. However, as the months passed, I acclimated, and the solace fed my true introverted tendencies, long-neglected and starving for attention.

After graduation, I was a coiled spring seeking to uncoil. A pervasive sense of emptiness and loneliness suddenly displaced the future-oriented optimism of my pre-doctoral journey. It was an abrupt, coup, contra-coup injury that left me very confused and sliding toward depression. Post doc crash? It felt like a postdoc apocalypse. After five years of intense study and an incredible graduation-day crescendo, I wondered what kind of denouement was just around the corner. In the days leading up to graduation, I kept telling myself how wonderful my new life and return to normalcy would be: I would go to the movies and enjoy eating meals in my kitchen. I managed to temporarily stave off the crash through long-overdue visits with old friends and binge-watching several years' worth of my favorite TV series. I even treated myself to a trip to the movies and an obligatory large popcorn drenched with butter.

My family and friends, whom I more or less neglected for four years, were brought back to center stage, and we started spending more time together. We did a tour of our favorite restaurants and resumed our tradition of sharing a weekly meal at my house. As life dictates, everyone had changed during my extended intellectual absence, but the process of rediscovering each other was magnificent.

Blissful days in safety continued.

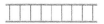

Then came a welcomed diversion, *the* project to fill time in my new post-doctoral life. My home had fallen into a sad state of disorganization during five years of doctoral study, so I threw myself into an intense home reorganization project that started in the front hall closet and concluded three months later in the garage. Order, freshness, and comfort were all re-established. No drawer, cabinet, or hidden area was untouched. I even managed to subjugate the kitchen's nefarious 'junk drawer.' With my whole family joining in, a huge multi-family garage sale followed, with the leftovers send to a local charity.

The nearly clean garage was the last area to be conquered. I purchased a pile driver for mounting brackets, my goal being to hang as much as I could on the walls so *my* garage would finally look as well-organized as those featured on TV home improvement shows.

That dream within grasp, I picked the afternoon of Thursday, September 29th, to complete the project and gathered the pile driver, screws, brackets, and extension ladder. "Take the time to gather all needed supplies before starting a procedure," I often told students. The pile driver looked like a drill but was intended to pound special concrete screws into the rigid masonry walls. It was cordless, light, and operated on a rechargeable lithium battery. Earlier that morning, another customer at the home improvement store was also shopping for a similar tool. He chatted with me, and although we agreed we weren't 'tool people,' we quickly came to the same conclusion: how hard could it be to operate such a small, lightweight, and cordless tool?

I had barely arrived home when I heard the doorbell ring. I was shocked, as this was the middle of a weekday, and wasn't sure anyone knew I was home. I peered out the window and saw my father, who said he could only stay a minute, as he was on his way to an appointment. He handed me a coupon, and I realized I could have saved five dollars on the tool I just purchased. *"Just my luck,"* I thought sarcastically. However, within a few minutes, it was indeed quite obvious there was absolutely nothing lucky about this day.

I was momentarily tempted to ask him to stay and help me—or at least take a look at what I was trying to accomplish—but for some reason, I was relieved he left so I could commence work on my project. I had come this far and wanted to see it through on my own. After all, I had just defended a dissertation, so this should be *easy*.

In retrospect, it seems hugely ironic my dad stopped by just before I mounted the ladder to hang the first bracket. He was the leader of our family's "Safety Team," who never missed an opportunity to give us some badly-needed coaching. "Clean that up, please. Don't leave that on the floor…someone might fall! Walk, don't run! Have somebody hold the ladder" are just some of the epithets I remember. His commentary was often framed within work experiences: we've had "50 days in safety…100 days in safety…*200 days in safety…*" He had accepted a buyout and retired in 1996, so it had been many years since he arrived home looking just a bit different when we knew the day's message was 'Zero Days in Safety.'

However, a semblance of familiarity remained in that for years after he wore his iconic pocket protector containing pens, note cards, and even the small screwdriver. The protector now included cards with important dates and other bits of information, including new terms and topics he wanted to research during his next trip to the library or the local historical society. Sometimes I wondered if he tried to initiate safety campaigns at those locations as well.

Smile.

Following my dad's quick departure for his next appointment, I can think of many things I would have done differently. Perhaps I would have asked him to stay so we could 'work as a team' or to just offer some simple advice; better yet, maybe he could have helped me find a way to work alone, but still safely. Unfortunately, a new entry would appear on the index card in his pocket on that day, but this time the entry was about me. Soon it would be his youngest child who caused that look of restrained horror on his face when one of his team was hurt and how I deeply regretted that.

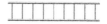

Tool in hand, I mounted the ladder and mapped out a strategy to hang the first bracket at the top of a wall near the ceiling. The 14-foot aluminum extension ladder had rubber feet, and I made sure they were firmly in place before my ascent. Safety check! I had lived in this house for over seven years now, totaling greater than 2,500 days in safety. That didn't even include the Days in Safety at the home or apartments before this one. Of course, 'little accidents' had happened, but nothing significant.

Just like at my childhood home, bad things didn't happen here, not in my world.

Bracket in place and fastener positioned, I hit the on the button and pushed…How hard could this be? I was looking forward to hanging about 20 brackets so my garage would simply be a marvel of organization and the envy of my neighbors.

I remember being so surprised by the rock-solid hardness of the masonry wall. After nearly a minute, there was still no progress, so I pushed harder and harder as the vibration and noise distracted my attention. I made a note to myself to tell the salesperson that this tool was not suitable for anything other than light household use and that I needed advice on which tool to purchase. This task shouldn't be so difficult. Maybe I should stop and take it back and buy something else. At least I could use the $5.00 coupon my dad had just given me...

WHOOOSSSHHH!!! BANG!!!!

PART II

ZERO DAYS IN SAFETY

CHAPTER 6

SOMETHING BAD HAPPENED HERE

Sometimes the bad things that happen in our lives put us directly on the path to the best things that will ever happen to us.
Nicole Reed

ONOMATOPOEIA.

That's what my 9th Grade honors English teacher called it. It took her a few minutes to convince us that such a ridiculous-sounding combination of letters was really a word. She had to retrieve the enormous Oxford Dictionary from the credenza next to her desk and read us the definition: a word that sounds just like the noise it describes, or something like that.

That impossible word was called into duty on just a few, potentially life-limiting seconds of my life. It was, and continues to be, very difficult for me to call forth an onomatopoeic word to describe that sound adequately. It was just a metallic noise resulting from a tall aluminum extension ladder hitting the concrete garage floor: an intense, highly pressured force, the air stirring from quick movement, and a vibration that seemed to last forever. More importantly, the noise meant the posting on my home's safety bulletin board would now have to be reset to zero.

Zero Days in Safety!

Something awful had just happened, right here in my own world.

Zero Days in Safety!

The ceiling's height in my garage is about 12 feet, and my face was positioned where the wall met the ceiling as I attempted to drill the first hole. In an instant, the aluminum extension ladder had fallen. As I pushed the pile driver with increasing levels of force against the masonry wall, I apparently didn't feel or notice the ladder's rubber feet slipping, which allowed it to slide down the wall with remarkable velocity and slam violently onto the concrete garage floor. A full 12-foot drop straight down experienced by an energized, though frustrated homeowner trying to use a new tool; a 12-foot transition from buoyantly optimistic post doc focused on home reorganization to dazed, broken, and semi-consciousness homeowner, all in less than a second.

A literal post doc crash indeed.

I heard that echoing metallic sound for months after, but it was never more vivid than in the first few moments after the accident. The sound, especially the vibration, became a part of me. Although it's challenging to describe, I felt it in my teeth for days afterward. I imagine it took less than one second for the ladder to slide down the wall and hit the floor. It happened so quickly there was no time to prepare. After the accident, several people asked me, "couldn't you have curled up in a ball to protect yourself?" or something like that. At that moment, I encountered an unthinkably overwhelming force, and I assured them there is no 'curling up in a ball' in a split-second confrontation with the beast known as gravity.

Because I was holding the drill, my arms were in front of me and absorbed much of the impact. I immediately knew something was terribly wrong with both of them, but my right arm seemed to be demanding the most attention. *"Please don't let me be hurt,"* I prayed silently, followed by audible incomprehensible moans and a series of thoughts of *"No, no, no, no...not my hands."*

I have always been a busy person, with hands in constant motion. The multi-tasker who types 125 words per minute. Betty, my former boss, commented on my performance evaluation that she "...had never met anyone who could juggle so many balls in the air at once." Over time, they transformed from a manager/administrator's hands into a Nurse's hands, still multi-tasking and, like most Nurses I knew, accomplishing an impossible number of acts of caring in one shift. In that instant, I knew my poor arms and hands had taken the brunt of a terrible injury. What had they done so wrong to receive such punishment?

Then again, since they had absorbed much of the impact, they helped shield my face and head. Nevertheless, my face had darted forward during the fall and glanced against something followed by a tearing sensation. Not a joyful sound like paper tearing on Christmas morning, but the dull, muted, sickening sound of living human tissue tearing accompanied by a prickly, tingling warm sensation. In an instant, I knew something very profound had happened to my body, my psyche, and my life.

That express trip from an elevation of 12 feet to ground zero was brief but transcendent, an invitation I would have declined had I had the chance. I was extraordinarily dazed and recalled effortlessly gliding to the bottom of Maslow's Hierarchy of Needs. One of the ladder's rungs must have pressed against my protruding abdomen and forced me to exhale, known in the vernacular as 'having the wind knocked out of you.' I focused solely on simply breathing. I was alive and nothing more.

My mind raced. *"Attention, students! So, this is what pressured thoughts must be like. I hoped I hadn't broken ribs…what was that called, a flail chest? When too many ribs are broken, the process of inspiration and expiration is interrupted, and sandbags must be applied. Had I punctured my abdomen, or worse yet, a lung? Please God, no. Who will help me? Focus. Breathe."* A few desperate but restorative breaths later, unbelievable, unbearable pain began to flow from every direction in my body. Fear, loss, and many other emotions and sensations simultaneously clamored for their fair share of my attention. I suddenly became aware of all parts of my body at once. Each one was checking in. I *could* breathe and, looking down, noticed I had not punctured my abdomen or chest. Good news? I hoped so.

One body part screamed more loudly than all the others, and I knew I would not emerge from this fall unscathed. Something was dreadfully wrong with my right arm. The pain was so overwhelming I transitioned into a brief episode of depersonalization as I looked down at my hand and examined it with detached fascination. I lectured about depersonalization every semester in psychiatric nursing; at that moment, I was experiencing it firsthand and somehow knew it. I looked at my right arm quizzically and studied it carefully, as though it belonged to someone else. As I have often discussed, the mind can disassociate itself from a body part or the entirety of one's being in an act of defiance, as if saying, "This isn't happening to me." I deliberately examined my right hand and wrist as though performing a clinical assessment. It was purple and very swollen, immediately becoming twice its normal size. It was also grossly misaligned, jutting off at about a 20-degree angle from my arm. Only when I attempted to move slightly did unspeakable pain, the apparent antidote to this episode of depersonalization, come out of hiding.

This accident certainly can't be good. I'm glad it's not happening to me.

But…it is…

Shame on you, Dr. Foley. A fall? Really. You were on the hospital's Falls Team for a long time. How could this happen?

Let's do a quick post-fall huddle:

- Non-skid footwear? Check.
- Area free from clutter? Check.
- Any medications interactions? No.
- Did you have someone hold the ladder for you? No, no, no! How foolish! Why not?

"Please don't chastise. That's no way to teach or inform, especially since nothing bad ever happened." At least not until today…a day where I found myself zero days in safety!

Zero days in safety!

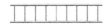

Although it was a beautiful day, I was suddenly freezing, as someone might feel in the middle of winter, or when they are stage-fright nervous, shocked, or terrified. Paradoxically, the only comfort in the first few moments after the accident was the sudden warmth flowing down my face until the stream trickled into my mouth and I tasted blood.

Badly shaken, my first semi-cogent thought was, *"Sir, what is your pain level on a scale of 1 to 10, 10 being the worst you have ever felt? Can you tell me the location and duration of the pain?"* I initially tried to push off the floor with my hands but was immediately thwarted by another round of tortured pain. Episode of depersonalization definitely resolved, I regained an acute focus on my condition.

I knew I was in my garage but was only aware of my physical being and not the least bit in touch with my surroundings. It's a sensation I can't fully describe other than assert when my mind reclaimed my body, I saw everything around me but only felt and sensed *me*. As much as I love God, my family, friends, pets, work, my students, and my life in general, this sudden change in circumstances forced me into a position where the only thing that possibly mattered was my very existence, a fact that even then made me feel uncharacteristically selfish.

I had to get out of that garage and get help.

The pain from other body parts flooded my consciousness. More unbelievable pain from my left arm, face, upper chest, right shoulder, and left knee joined forces with the pain in my right arm, forming a tsunami. My left hand and left arm hurt terribly, but not as much as my right hand. Rather than acute pain, they instead felt strangely weak. My stomach hurt. My legs hurt. My head hurt. The pain continued to grow, and I just froze. Robbed of the luxury of an initial numbing shock, I attempted to rationalize. *"Don't move, and maybe it will go away...you know...like when you stub your toe on a piece of furniture...it's unbearable at first but then mostly goes away, settling itself into a dull tolerable throb. Maybe this won't be so bad after all".*

Unfortunately, it did not get better but seemed to get even worse.

This *really* wasn't good.

The pain was in a tug of war with the warmth flowing down my face. I spit blood onto the garage floor several times. As I looked down, blood dropped from my chin and dotted the floor, and I stared at it quizzically. I had just installed a new garage floor, and now this section looked like a crime scene. *"You'll never get it clean,"* I told myself. *"Mom always said blood is one of the hardest stains to treat. What will she say when she sees this?"*

Driven by the pain, I instinctively turned to my Faith. *"Ok, God,"* I thought, *"you have my full, undivided attention. You're obviously trying to tell me something. What will I learn from this? Have I neglected you over these past years of doctoral pursuit and career growth?"* Memories of church, Bible passages, old hymns, and words of inspiration flooded me. The trauma released my Faith, and I chose to hold fast, whether this was the end of my life or the beginning of a long recovery.

"Ok, God, what is all this about?"

Note to self: be sure to remind every student and practicing Nurse that a patient's spiritual resources are a potent source of strength. In addition to the articles on spirituality you share with students, you will now have a powerful, highly personal story to tell.

My enduring framework of Faith refused to entertain the thought that this accident might be the end. I knew I was in big trouble, but I would survive.

Buckle up and hang on, Nurse.

I sat nearly motionless in that garage for approximately 45 minutes, wanting to speak but only managing a chant-like "ahh…ahh" over and over in perfect sync with wave after wave of pain. I realized I was attempting to speak, but the pain was so unbearable all I could do was slowly rock back and moan in a rhythmic series of self-comforting movements. I tried again to push off from the floor with my left arm, knowing my right arm in its 20-degree deviant state would be of no assistance. Despite its weakness, my left arm was just strong enough, and I sat upright.

In my typical pragmatic fashion, I forged an action plan consisting of three complex tasks: get off the floor, get back in the house, and call for help. I scooted over to a shelving unit, anchored myself with my chin, and used my abdominal and leg muscles to stand. The shelving unit began to tip during the process, but I paused while the unit righted itself and then slowly, carefully got up. Another accident was avoided.

"Does that near-miss count, or can I still take credit for about an hour in safety? No, I don't think that counts at this point…"

Now on my feet, I shuffled slowly and deliberately across the garage floor's 25-foot expanse to push the button on the kitchen's entry door with my cheek. Unfortunately, when the button is pressed, the handle must be engaged to open the door. I tried several times with my left hand but couldn't do it. My hand was just too weak. If I could just make it into the house, maybe I could sit at the kitchen table…get some ice…. lay down… perhaps this would all go away. I did not want to call for help. Instead, I desired to keep this event, this accident, a secret for as long as possible, just dreading the next steps.

"Nurse, this is not going to go away. You need to get help. Stop stalling and get help...now." I opened the garage door by hitting a large, user-friendly wall-mounted button with my nose, shuffled into the driveway, and screamed. No more polite, compensatory "ahh...ahhs." I found my voice and screamed loud, desperate, and agonizing cries for help. After suffering in near silence for nearly an hour, the sound of my screams startled me. I yelled again and again, and each time I did, the noise seemed to aggravate the pain. I just wanted to sit still, be quiet, and make the whole world stop, but silence would not summon help, and that's what I needed.

I lived in a development with homes only 50 feet apart, so certainly, *someone* would hear me. It was the middle of the afternoon, and I expected a neighbor's front door to open, or better yet, someone emerge from their back patio, see my distress, and come running toward me with their cell phone in hand. Incredibly, no one *was* home, so I was left standing there by myself. After seven years of living in a neighborhood of retirees and stay-at-home moms, I can say with some degree of certainty that someone is *always* home, but not now. There was just me, my 20-degree deviant right hand, dripping blood, the pain, my screams, and sheer terror all standing there in the middle of the driveway in one big discordant mess. Since I not only teach—but truly believe—a patient's spiritual resources can be beneficial in times of crisis, I can say with certainty God was there too.

I'm so glad He was.

I struggled back into the garage and once again used my nose in several vain attempts to open the entry door from the garage into the kitchen. This time I used my left little finger to pull hard when I depressed the button and was surprised when the door finally sprung open. Stepping into the kitchen, I saw my cell phone sitting just a few feet away in the entry hall, and I used my semi-functional left little finger to dial my sister. We have always been close, and I knew this accident would profoundly affect such a sensitive human being. I had no choice but to call her and cringed when she answered the phone immediately.

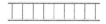

When we were growing up, my sister Ellen was a 'candy striper' volunteer at our local community hospital. She dutifully fulfilled her hours, earned her candy striper cap, and became close with Sister D., a nun who ran the volunteer program. Sister D. even went so far as to call our home one hot summer afternoon to ask my mother if she would please encourage my sister to enter the hospital's Practical Nursing Program upon graduation from high school. "Sister D., thank you very much for your suggestion, but I can't do that. My daughter faints at the sight of blood." Amid smiles and soft laughter, my mother continued, "as much as she likes being a candy striper, she's just not cut out to be a Nurse. I agree with you. She would make a great Nurse, but it's just not possible."

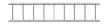

Faints at the site of blood.

Well, sorry to break the news to you, sis, but I suspect there's much blood to be seen here today. Although I had mirrors all over my home, it never occurred to me to look into one of them. I'm glad I didn't because I'm sure I was a mess. I hoped the passage of 40 years had changed her faint-at-the-site-of-blood response—otherwise we would both be in trouble.

When she answered, I managed to transcend the physical and emotional realms to sound surprisingly calm and casual. The sound of my everyday speaking voice was startling, even more than the sound of my shrieks.

In retrospect, I should have called 911 and would certainly advise anyone else in my situation to do the same. Falls from ladders can be debilitating and even life-threatening, requiring immediate intervention. Despite my physical injuries, I rationalized that a potential head trauma wasn't a concern, at least according to my depersonalized garage floor self-assessment.

Why?

I stood there and reasoned that, as long as I went to a specific hospital seven miles from my home, my teacher's health insurance would pay 100% of usual and customary charges *with no co-insurance and no deductible.* See…I *must* be cognitively intact! The hospital is most easily accessed from secondary roads but not via the freeway. The trip would take about a half-hour at best.

An ambulance trip would more than likely have to be paid out-of-pocket and was so expensive. *An on-the-spot cost-benefit analysis of my own transportation and follow-up emergency care at a time like this?*

Yes, I must be cognitively intact.

I carefully mapped out our route in my mind, whispering the names of each street as my mind perused an imaginary map. Indeed, if I could process all of this information, my brain's executive functions were intact, and I *must not have hit my head*. I resolved that since it was the middle of the day, traffic would be light, and my plan for medical assistance sans economic devastation might work—provided my sister didn't faint.

Yet despite assumptions of a cognitively intact mind, I should have called 911 and urge everyone to do the same.

After a brief moment of 'what are you up to this afternoon' pleasantries, I launched into carefully measured discourse, driven by intense pain; I was concerned I might be going into shock. She knew me too well and sensed something had happened. "David, what's wrong?" she called urgently into the phone.

"I need you to listen to me very carefully and remain calm. I've been in a terrible accident in the garage. I broke both of my arms and cut myself; I'm sure my face is involved. There's a lot of blood, so please bring a blanket to cover the seats. I don't want to get blood all over your new car. It's very, very bad, and I may have other broken bones, cuts, and internal injuries. Please don't be upset when you see me."

To her credit, she remained calm and only inserted an occasional "OK" as I spoke. The sister who could not be a Nurse because she faints at the site of blood and thus thwarted Sister D's vision for her life held herself together and came through like a real pro—but then fell apart later in the day when no one was looking.

Perhaps she could be a Nurse after all.

Although she lives only 3 ½ miles away, a 10-15-minute drive even in moderate traffic, the wait seemed endless. I somehow got outside and waited for her in the driveway, hiding behind the expanse of my beautiful magnolia tree. I heard a car coming and saw the next-door neighbor pull into her driveway. Then I noticed the neighbor across the street pull into her driveway and start retrieving groceries from the trunk.

Now they come home.

My rescue plan fell quickly into place, however. Just as both neighbors disappeared into their homes, I saw my sister's shiny new black car appear in the distance and then glide to a stop in my driveway. Only then did my legs, the only parts of me that seemed strong, falter just a bit. I grabbed for the flimsy support of my Magnolia Tree's lower branches and called out to her. To her credit, she remained expressionless as she efficiently wrapped me into a blanket and walked us toward her car. Nursing instructors often say, "a Nurse's facial expression should never convey their true feelings, no matter how difficult the patient's condition."

"Yes, sis, maybe you can be a Nurse after all."

Ellen opened the door, and I carefully lowered myself into the car. As I swung my legs around, she reached out and touched my grossly displaced right hand. I screamed loud and long. "I'm so sorry," she said, and I simply replied, "It's ok. Let's go. Hurry." We never made eye contact nor said anything meaningful to each other during the short but endless trip to the hospital. Although I had minimal control of my arms, any movement was so painful I could not reach up and pull the visor down to inspect my appearance in the mirror. My sister gently but firmly denied my requests to pull it down for me.

We both knew her reasons for doing so.

I recall her sympathetic side glances when I winced each time the car hit a bump or, worse yet, a pothole. Although she told me several times to sit back and try to be as quiet as possible, our destination was outside her mental map, and I needed to be her navigator. Our destination was designated as a Level 1 Trauma Center, and in fact, part of the area's healthcare folklore was 'if you ever get hurt, be sure to go there. They do trauma the best.'

When we finally and mercifully entered the hospital's campus, we passed the long-term care facility where my elderly maternal aunt has lived for the past 12 years. She suffered a head injury at the age of 14, and from that moment on, the older members of the family said she was "never quite the same." Although she went on to get married, have children, and work at a local business, the specter of that head injury subsequent mental health diagnosis haunted her. She began frequently falling in her early 60s and had to be placed in a moderate level of care nursing home at the age of only 69. *"I'm so young. I'm glad I wasn't killed, but will I end up living here? I hope not. Does that make me a snob, not wanting to be hurt and live in this long-term care facility at the age of 50? We always said it was such a nice facility, but that is for her, not me, right?"*

Right! Did I hit my head and would now have a head injury that would haunt me for decades? I didn't think so. Logic roared back that if I had, I would still be lying on the garage floor. I must have hit my head on *something*, hence the trauma to my face. As the scenery drifted by, I performed a quick neuro assessment on myself:

- **Person:** Dr. David Foley
- **Place:** My sister's car
- **Time:** September 29th about 2:30 pm
- **Circumstance**: on my way to the area's best Emergency Room for trauma injuries related to a fall from a ladder.
- Yes, I was 'alert and oriented X 4' and, with that robust validation, acknowledged it was time to fight! I was going to the hospital, but from there, I would go *home*.

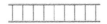

"Is this it? Are we here?" my sister's words summoned me back from my daydreams. God bless her, but a *huge* red and white sign directly in front of the car screamed 'Emergency Room Drop-Off.' Under other circumstances, I would have made some snappy come-back in true brother-sister fashion, but on this day, all I could say was "yes...go." I tried to use my hand to motion but cried out. How quickly I had forgotten. The pain caused me to turn my head, and despite my wincing, I noticed I was face to face with a second red and white sign that screamed even louder, "Wrong Way. Do Not Enter." Oh no! The emergency room's drop-off was a circular driveway, and I had just told her to enter the wrong way.

An older man dressed in a security guard's outfit burst through the automatic doors and ran toward her car, waving his hand in a fiercely dismissive gesture. "You're going the wrong way," I read his lips more than heard the words.

"Help my brother, help my brother, *help my brother*," I called out, supplying my sister with the words I was afraid she couldn't speak. "Help my brother," my sister yelled when he appeared at the passenger door's window yelling, "You're going the wrong way." He talked to her but locked eyes with me as she cried out again, "please help my brother." I wasn't sure what he saw, but his face instantly turned from anger to concern as he opened the door. "Can he walk? Hurry, miss, can he walk?"

He? It was the first of many, many times I would be referred to as "he," a manner I always advised my students to avoid. "Does the 'he' (or 'she') have *a name?*" I would ask them. I never learned *his* name but granted him a dispensation at that moment. This afternoon was not the time for etiquette or discussion about the importance of therapeutic communication. Temporary residence at the bottom of Maslow's Hierarch of Needs supersedes such social and professional conventions.

"Please help my brother," I heard Ellen say again. I don't think she heard the security guard's question, and for the first time, I saw her fall apart just a bit. The gravity of the situation finally showed on her face with wide, opened eyes, tears flowing, and hair not in its usually pristine state. She had dropped everything and came running after my call. I often advise patients and their families of the need to just "fall apart" as a means to dissipate stress and regain a measure of control. *"Please, sis,"* I thought, *"don't' fall apart just yet. Wait until I'm in the hospital, then park your car and make it to the waiting room. Then you can fall apart. We're not quite there yet."*

Just then, I saw a woman dressed in scrubs finish helping a patient into the car next to us and simultaneously saw the driver of that car look at our vehicle quizzically, knowing we were going the wrong way and blocking his egress.

Oh no, please. There's no time for 'who has the right-of-way now.'

I summoned all my strength and once again used my highly useful left pinky to open the car door, then swung my legs out. "Wait," I called to the woman in scrubs. "Help me!" Her eyes met mine, and her face also dissolved into concern and as she rushed closer to me and I saw the letters RN clearly emblazoned on her name tag. Our eyes momentarily made contact, and we had a long, meaningful conversation without saying a word.

I now had silent confirmation from an RN colleague that this was not good. I never said goodbye to my sister. She is so sensitive, and I'm sure she would have benefitted from at least a moment of reassurance. My natural impulse to survive, coupled with unspoken confirmation of my circumstances by another RN, pushed me with a singular focus toward help and away from civility. It was only when I tried to stand that I realized I was weak, fragile, and possibly going into shock; only waves of unbelievable pain kept me alert. I noticed this Nurse carefully lock the wheelchair brakes and saw her stoic, tempered reaction when I screamed out as she touched my arm to help me into the wheelchair. I was quite embarrassed to scream in front of this new RN colleague.

How could I be here? How could I let this happen? What will I do now in this unfamiliar territory known as 'zero days in safety'?

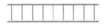

I cannot describe what happened, but over the next few moments and through a haze of chaotic, muddled thoughts, I realized an unprecedented opportunity was at hand. "Everything life sends you is an opportunity," a former mentor said. "Rise up and face it with courage and dignity. If it becomes overwhelming, crouch down and let the chaos pass. What will be left behind is opportunity." Like my father, I often wrote down meaningful phrases, and that is one quote that I have stored in a safe place. Upon that recollection, I decided to transport myself from this terrible physical experience into an intellectual journey of discovery. Life. Opportunity. Rise up. Face it with courage. Dignity. Overwhelming. Crouch down. Let chaos pass.

I had been, among other roles, a Nurse, Nurse Educator, Nurse Manager, Director of Operations, Program Director, Hospital Administrator, Systems Analyst, Compliance Surveyor, Consultant, and Performance Improvement Council team member, but never a patient—not like this at least. I had only existed on the other side, in roles that sought to improve the quality of the patient care experience. Now it was my turn to have my own experience.

As my mind continued to race, I somehow transported myself outside my body into a highly intellectual space, one where there was no pain, no broken bones, no tissue damage, and no blood—only rich opportunity. *"This is good,"* I reasoned, *"use this experience as a patient to gain perspective to help others and educate students."* What interesting things would I see, smell, feel, and experience in this role of the patient? I often said once you have been in nursing, you just know too much, and it ruins the patient experience for you and your loved ones. My hunch told me a whole bunch of assertions were about to be destroyed.

Here goes...

PART III

ZERO DAYS IN SAFETY: CARE IN THE TRAUMA SERVICE

CHAPTER 7

UNDERCOVER

Quality is never an accident. It is always the result of high intention, sincere effort, intelligent direction, and skillful execution. It represents the wise choice of many alternatives, the cumulative experience of many masters of craftsmanship.
William A. Foster

FROM THE MOMENT the emergency department's automatic doors whisked open with perfect symmetry, I resolved to take in every sight, sound, and experience in an homage to my former, current, and future students. I often told my classes about every Nurse's 'suitcase of stories' that starts out very small but quickly expands with every new patient interaction and clinical scenario. When I graduated from my pre-licensure program, my virtual suitcase was so small I could carry it on my key chain—like one of those little plastic suitcases containing a rain bonnet my mom used to buy on the strip at Niagara Falls. However, after many years of practice, it had become a heavy, unwieldy trunk, and frankly, I wish I could give some of those stories back. Nevertheless, I celebrated my cache of experiences as the best source of information for classroom illustrations and often coped with challenging situations by reminding myself they would make remarkable case studies one day.

Despite these noble intentions, as the wheelchair surged forward, my thoughts became an unintelligible mess as I rode waves of hot, fluid pain. I coped just a bit by imagining my virtual support system: family, friends, colleagues, students, and of course, my Faith. I pictured all of them comprising my 'lines of defense' that were pierced by this injury and begging to mend. Time to rally my troops, Dr. Betty Neuman!

Albeit virtually, they were all there right there in front of me and at the ready to provide comfort and reassurance. Memories flashed by in rapid succession, and I tapped into them to remain in an intellectual space where the pain became bearable through the power of guided imagery. I visualized myself disappearing through an escape hatch away from this terrible experience and embarking on a fact-finding mission that would one day promote meaningful learning, discussion, and reflection.

I resolved that for now, I would not tell anyone I was a Nurse, former hospital administrator, or college professor.

I would go undercover.

How intriguing...

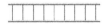

I straddled the divide between my tortured physical being and bruised psyche. This absolutely could not be happening to me, at least not now. Each movement brought pain and more racing thoughts: "*no, you are not a patient, you are a Nurse Educator—a doctorally-prepared one at that and with so much to do.*" I winced and grunted softly, even as the wheelchair transitioned from the exterior walkway to glide over the smoothness of the Emergency Department's terrazzo floor.

Perhaps I could demonstrate my cognitive 'intactness' through a simple prosocial act of initiating a conversation. "What's your name?" I asked this RN. "Erica. What happened to you, sir?" Nurse Erica's disembodied voice asked from behind. It was bizarre to have someone speak to my back while we were moving at such velocity. I often reinforced the importance of mindfulness with students: stop, feet planted on the ground, face the patient, make direct eye contact, smile, and only then speak. However, I acquiesced those principles must often be suspended during times of acute crises, and this was indeed a crisis. Mindful, therapeutic communication would have to wait, at least for now.

"Fall from ladder" was all I could mutter to my new RN colleague. Actually, I hadn't fallen from a ladder. The ladder collapsed, but that was too much to explain, so "fall from ladder" seemed most manageable. I wasn't sure if Nurse Erica had heard me, so I repeated a little louder, "I fell from a ladder in my garage." *"Tell her you are a Nurse,"* my id-driven emotions screamed, *"maybe you will get some extra attention…sympathy…better care".* As self-serving as it sounds, that's what I thought, and to be honest, I wonder how many other Nurse colleagues would have thought the same thing.

"You fell from a ladder? How high were you? Did you hit your head?" she called out as we entered the impossibly noisy milieu of the emergency room's main lobby. The abrupt change was painful. The noise hurt. *"Nurse Erica, please don't ask me to talk more. I'm in such pain. Can't you just read my mind instead?"* "About 12 feet and no" was all I could reply.

I remember seeing so many people move in and out of my field of gaze as we proceeded with the incredible velocity created by Nurse Erica wheeling her unexpected new patient with great purpose and energy. A woman sitting in the waiting room absently-mindedly glanced from the TV, made eye contact with me, and then stared at me wide-eyed. Since her facial expression *did* convey her true feelings, I decided she must not be a Nurse. The man sitting with her avoided his gaze and looked down at the floor, so I decided he must not be a Nurse. "Hello," I said rather pleasantly, but he looked intently away and said nothing.

Each time I spoke, I felt my upper lip flapping in a somewhat unnatural manner. I could only imagine what the waiting room's occupants were seeing. A woman sat with two small children, one of whom was playing quietly while the other stared directly at me. She picked up the child and gave her a big hug, a sudden, affectionate act from a caring mother who didn't want her child to witness something grotesque. I was touched by the mother's protective action but realized it meant bad news was on its way.

"How is your shift going, Erica?" I asked, and she quickly replied, "fine," as she punched the wall plate with a closed fist to activate the automatic door which separated the waiting room from the treatment area. *So terse, Nurse Erica. Are you unfriendly or just on a mission?* "I'm glad one of us is doing fine. I've had better days, as you can see." Would she notice my wit and sarcasm as more signs of an intact cognition? My plan was already forming. *They will see how good I am and I'll be treated and released* because I want to get out of here as quickly as possible and go home where nothing bad ever happened—well, almost never.

But don't forget, Nurse Foley. You're now in Zero Days in Safety....

More people, mostly patients, moved in and out of view as pieces of equipment and rooms swept past. A gentleman in the hallway didn't look good. His skin was ashen, and he appeared to be in respiratory distress. The head of his bed was elevated, and he was wearing a mask inhaling a fine mist, which I presumed was a respiratory treatment. We made eye contact, and so far, he was the only person who didn't react. We just exchanged sympathetic glances, making an unspoken bond between two people who weren't doing very well right now. *"Try to relax, sir, and just take some long, deep breaths. That medicine is going to help you,"* I said in my mind, but that was the Nurse in me speaking, and I wasn't here for that. I was a patient here to receive advice and care myself.

A young boy, possibly age 7, was sitting on another bed crying and receiving comfort from his mother. His cries got louder, and I noticed some casting supplies nearby. *"A broken bone for you too, young man? As soon as you get your cast on, you'll be going home. Hang in there, ok?"*

Who do you think you're fooling, Nurse Foley? You're just saying that to make yourself feel better because you want to go home too.

Nurse Erica stopped very briefly, perhaps 10 seconds, to speak with a registration clerk. "Going to Bay 1. Fall from Ladder. Obvious deformity right hand. Facial laceration."

"I have my ID and insurance cards in my wallet...I know the drill." I smiled pleasantly, but my smile felt contorted, asymmetrical, and burned with pain. Although I didn't touch it, my nose felt numb, and I decided I must have really injured my face.

"No time for that now sir, she'll get all that from you later," Nurse Erica said not unpleasantly but very matter-of-factly. "I am a 'Select' patient, and I do have my insurance card," I called out to the clerk as she quickly disappeared out of view.

Be sure to remind them you should be covered at 100% with no coinsurance and no deductible. That's why you didn't call 911 and came here by car. Can you imagine what the bill would have been if you went anywhere else? Yes, I'm in-network...

No, Dr. Foley, you should have called 9-1-1 instead. How foolish!

Erica's hands stiffened on the handles of the wheel-chair, and once again, we were on our way. I felt the renewed energy of this caregiver as she pushed the wheel-chair. It traveled through the handles, and her strength and purpose comforted me. I sensed she wouldn't be moving this quickly unless she thought it was serious but was reassured by our serendipitous meeting in the driveway and her take-charge approach. Her swift action meant care was on the way.

The cool air hitting my face as we sped down the hallway seemed strangely refreshing; on another day, it might have felt quite good, but this was not like any other day. The trip seemed very long, but I remembered this hospital, one of only three in the metropolitan area des-ignated as a Level I Trauma Center, had recently rebuilt its Emergency Department, which was now housed in this enormous building. I realized this was the hospital where I previously worked as a Director of Operations and fell in love with the profession of nursing. Over the years, I kept tabs on new developments through a dear friend who still worked there.

I meant to return one day to visit but not like this....
Glancing around, I was impressed by not only the Emergency Department's sheer size but by the number of people receiving care. There was a patient on a cart in every room. Good for patient volume and statistics, but even better for revenue, especially if the patients have commercial insurance like me.

Don't be so elitist or conceited...patients have a right to privacy and care, regardless of the circumstances or their type of insurance...you should know better! My superego screamed, but my id roared back: *Fool. All of this nonsense is one big coping mechanism to help with the pain. Stop trying to impress. We are hurting right now, and you know it!* My ego stayed out of it and simply pouted somewhere in the recesses of my psyche.

We turned a corner, and I noted the décor had changed, especially the color scheme and the signage. The word 'trauma,' with all its implied connotations, was everywhere. *Trauma? Yes, trauma...and don't act surprised, you know where are going* my id, ego, and super-ego called out in an unprecedented showing of unity. Groups of staff hung in clusters by small Nurse's stations that moved past me one after another as the wheelchair moved swiftly. I couldn't help but notice their stares, but none of these trained professionals averted their gaze or turned away. They looked straight at me and were not shocked a bit, so clearly, something captured their attention. *Oh yes, the blood.* It had dried on my face and lips, which felt very sticky in some areas and tight in others. Looking down, I noticed my shirt was covered with blood as well. *Was all that blood from an auto accident, gunshot, stabbing…. What must they think? Who cares what they think? It's time to get help.*

Trauma Bay 4, Trauma Bay 3, Trauma Bay 2…

As I was whisked into Trauma Bay 1, I accepted I was not just visiting the Emergency Department, but the *Trauma Center*. Really sick, injured people are taken to the Trauma Center. I recalled from my administrative training that the Trauma Service is very costly and labor-intensive and more than likely considered one of the most expensive points in the critical care continuum. Look at all the staff waiting. Were they all here for me? Think of the labor costs involved with…

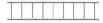

I started to lose the ability to navigate the space between my stealthily-contrived intellectual space and physical injuries. It was nice while it lasted, but walls were tumbling down, and reality was swiftly approaching. My sympathetic nervous system was earning its keep maintaining my fight response; my respirations increased and my heartbeat faster and faster. There was fight, but from this experience, there would be no flight. I just wanted to go home but knew I had to stay and face what was to come.

Thoughts and images surged through my mind at an overwhelming, unprecedented speed. So this is what racing thoughts are like? As I taught in my Psychiatric-Mental Health Nursing class, I knew racing thoughts are often associated with acute mania or episodes of severe panic. My mind was moving so quickly that I was aware of my thoughts' totality but simply could not get a 'fix" on any of them.

I'm supposed to be at work tomorrow. Who will get the mail? The food will spoil in my refrigerator. We have a subcommittee meeting scheduled to discuss some important business regarding the University. I also have some time blocked out to finish a publication. My cats need to be fed. I hope I locked my car. Tomorrow's a Friday as well. I wish I had cleaned my house. Only one more day until the weekend and its promise of some rest, maybe even a movie. Mow the lawn...

Faster and faster they went until they were a jumbled mess. In psychiatric nursing, we look for themes within a patient's thoughts. Paranoid. Grandiose. Depressed. The overall themes of *my* racing thoughts were loss, fear of dependence, and fear of inaction. Why had this happened to me, a newly-graduated PhD with so many plans?

The single event of ascending a ladder in my garage ended an outstanding track record of thousands of days in safety, a most generous run that helped me create a firmly engrained personal narrative of safety and security. Although I had worked in health care settings for years, I worked only in the role of caregiver, a luxury that allowed me to glide effortlessly in and out of complex, often tragic patient scenarios, knowing it was *them* and not *me*. At the end of each workday, I went home to comfort and safety, but today I was in a 'Zero Days in Safety' scenario, and now I must accept that.

"Racing thoughts. Simply put, the mind can't keep up with itself. Racing thoughts can be very frightening for many patients, especially when they are first diagnosed." *Well said, Professor Foley, only this time, the 'they' are you. Are you scared?*

Yes. Oh yes.

Interestingly, fear of pain, needles, procedures, or anything else associated with the medical aspects of this untoward trip to the Emergence Department was not foremost in my mind. Instead, I was experiencing a sense of anticipatory grief over the loss of independence, exacerbated by the terror of missing work and being perceived as irresponsible. What would people think if I couldn't show up for work on Monday? Who would take care of the house, my parents, the cats, the lawn, my student advisees…..?

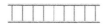

From a young age, I was the 'responsible one,' learning the "Citizenship" and "Most Dependable" awards in the 2nd and 6th grades, respectively. A strong sense of duty was a big part of my identity, continuing to grow throughout my lifetime. Arriving to work at 4:00 am (without being asked, mind you) to help with Environment of Care Rounds. Never the drinker, always the designated driver. Never the laggard, consistently the producer, the leader on doctoral group projects so my colleagues would *know* I was carrying my weight and could 'cut it.'

As a brand new doctoral graduate, my new responsibilities grew to include many more opportunities to demonstrate both commitment and respectability: writing, teaching, research, leadership, and mentoring. Further progress in any of these areas must now wait. Someone else would now have to be the responsible one for now. Self-loathing crept in—maybe I couldn't cut it after all.

Idiot. You went almost seven years once without missing a day of work at your last job and received an award for perfect attendance. There certainly wouldn't be any special awards for perfect attendance—or dependability—in the near future. So many lost opportunities on the horizon…

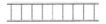

The wheelchair made its abrupt right turn into Trauma Bay 1, and at that moment, my gaze focused on two people standing behind the desk: a Nurse and a Physician. Through the haze of pain, I assumed the woman dressed in scrubs was the Nurse, and the man dressed in a crisp long white coat was the Physician. *"The person wearing the white coat must be the doctor, right?"* my thoughts raced. Was it sexist of me, an educated man, to think that as I sat in a wheelchair trapped in a maze of pain? I make such a point of teaching about creating nursing identities free from gender bias. Were the trauma and pain causing my true colors to show? I hoped not, especially as co-chair of the School of Nursing's Diversity and Inclusion Committee….

"What's going on?" the man in the white lab coat called out?

"I'm sorry to interrupt, doctor, but as you can see, there's actually a lot going on!" I screamed without saying a word.

He was wearing thick glasses that made his eyes look impossibly small. How could he ever see without them? But then again, they went so well with his white coat, creating the perfect image of medical intellectualism. I closed my eyes for a few moments, eventually opening them to find his face quite near mine. It was quite startling to see his tiny, liquid blue eyes scrutinizing me. "Open your eyes, sir," he spoke, and I smelled something on his breath. Fast food. Grease and something spicy. They must have been eating lunch. I suddenly felt very nauseous and closed my eyes to quell the urge to vomit. "I'm closing my eyes because I feel extremely nauseous. Just in case, you better stand back for a moment, doctor...or Nurse, or...."

"Fall from ladder. Obvious deformity right hand. Facial laceration" Nurse Erica spoke with terse authority to the whole room and then turned to speak to a new woman dressed in scrubs that matched the color she was wearing. As if anticipating their next question, Nurse Erica called out, "I don't know anything other than that. I was discharging another patient and ran into him in the parking lot. He's answering basic questions."

Basic questions, Nurse Erica? I can answer much more than just basic questions if you will only ask me. I know all the Presidents in order, am great at trivia, and would love to tell you a bit about my dissertation over coffee sometime.

"Can he stand?" the new woman asked Nurse Erica. I had gotten used to Nurse Erica's voice in the past few minutes, and this new voice startled me for a moment. Another Nurse with whom I must interact as a patient. *New Nurse, please be therapeutic, ok?* "He stood and got into the wheelchair by himself," Nurse Erica replied as she moved me closer to the gurney, applied the wheelchair's breaks, and moved the footrests out of the way. Several sets of eyes fell on me as everyone paused for just a few moments to watch me stand and transfer.

"I will show them what I can do so we can stop this nonsense, and I can go home." Once again, using my prized core muscles, I prepared to stand but thought: *"He. He. He. The second time in five minutes someone has referred to me in the third person. I hope there isn't a third instance because now I'm considering this a teachable moment. Please speak to me directly. I'm here and am able to respond. Do you refer to all your patients by their pronouns? He, she, they…."*

I took a moment to scrutinize this new woman's ID carefully, saw the welcomed RN insignia, and noted her name was Vivian. "Vivian, I can stand if you'll give me a moment," quite intentionally using her name in the spirit of my Dale Carnegie Training. Would *she* be impressed? Apparently, she could have cared less that I either knew her name or tried to impress her. I could almost sense their impatience as Erica and Vivian intently watched while I stood up, turned, and then sat on the gurney. *See, I'm not a trauma patient after all,* denial screamed. *Look at all the things I can do! I pleasantly greet people, address them by name, and can stand and transfer by myself. I might be a patient, but certainly not a trauma patient. I know I need help, but I belong in another part of the continuum of care—not here. Maybe I could go to the regular ED or be treated in the office…*

Erica made eye contact with me one last time and said, "Good luck, sir," before she grabbed the handles of the wheelchair, turned, and quickly left Trauma Bay 1. Just like that, she was gone. I became pretty attached to Nurse Erica and her efficiency in the less than 5 minutes I had almost been her patient. I was very sorry to see her go. I knew our meeting in the parking lot fell into the fantastic 'right place at the right time Divine intervention' category, and I celebrated the value of her unflinching offer of assistance. I later learned Nurses in the Emergency Department are assigned to teams and that Nurse Erica didn't even work in the Trauma area. Nevertheless, she made eye contact with me in the driveway, instinctively knew what I needed, and sprang into action to get me assistance as quickly as possible. As a seasoned Nurse, she demonstrated advocacy by adopting me as her patient right on the spot.

So well done, Nurse Erica. If you were one of my students in clinicals, I would give you an A+ and tell you to please be sure to use this case for one of your care plans—I think it would make for interesting reading. Will you please complete a reflective journal as well? I am also giving you a 'heads up' that you would be presenting in our post-conference, so take some time to get ready.

Bye, wonderful Nurse Erica. Now let's see what Nurse Vivian can do.

Just as Nurse Vivian turned to greet me, the energy level in the room surged as a crowd of people swarmed around. "Lay down, sir," said the bespectacled man in a white coat in an authoritative niceties-can-wait-until-later voice, so I swung my legs up and laid down. For some reason, I didn't like him. No logical explanation, as I knew he was here to help me, but I just didn't like him.

"OK, class, here's an interesting topic: negative transference, or the unexplained negative feelings the patient has toward the caregiver, usually resulting from some unresolved subconscious conflict or prior negative experience." I wondered of whom he reminded me. It must be one of the Physicians I worked with in the past. Very Freudian, but these caregivers certainly weren't worried about anything Freudian. They were working only within the medical realm and wanted to assess my physical status immediately.

Now flat on the examination table, I felt very dizzy and wondered if I was going into shock. I was surrounded by people who were calling out vital signs, assessing my pupillary response, and just trying to ensure my life wasn't in imminent danger. I think I had held it together for as long as I could and knew I couldn't "just hang in there" any longer. *I guess you belong here after all.*

Guided imagery. *Just close your eyes and take deep breaths. You're on that cozy beach in Bermuda. You had such a great time there. Feel the warmth of the sun on your face and the delightful sensation of the sand under your feet.*

Guided imagery can be so helpful to promote relaxation, even in the most challenging circumstances. Everyone has a favorite place they like to go, so go, Nurse Foley. I pretended the exam light was the sun and recalled when my best friend and I searched for shells on the beach. I did, and it was a glorious journey, even for just a few minutes. We brought some shells home, and they are still on display in my study...

Excruciating pain, an unwelcomed intruder, summoned me back from my imaginary vacation: someone had inadvertently bumped into my right arm. I managed to keep it perfectly still for the few minutes during the wheelchair ride and transfer and had just settled into a cold, clammy sense of comfort on the beach in Bermuda. As I screamed out in pain, I admit I had some very unkind thoughts for the person who bumped into my injured extremity. I couldn't believe such pain was possible as tears involuntarily streamed down my face.

The man spoke to me again, and I momentarily ignored him. *Class selective ignoring can be very useful when trying to extinguish a maladaptive behavior.* Unfortunately, he was neither doing nor saying anything maladaptive. He was just doing his job and trying to be helpful. The pain was preventing me from offering a response.

The fact that I just didn't like him or his bedside manner made matters worse. Then again, I worked in Psychiatric Nursing with its glorious focus on therapeutic communication. He worked in a different part of the hospital and resultantly had a demeanor and communication skill set very different from mine. Nevertheless, his style supported his work and mission in the Trauma Unit, and I knew that.

In my Psychiatric-Mental Health Nursing course, I teach students about the wonder of slowly peeling back the layers of an onion, a metaphor for breaking through to 'difficult' patients. Would I expect any caregiver working in the Trauma Unit to have the skills, ability, or desire to engage me with such gentle therapeutic communication? Probably not. They were there to save lives, and there simply wasn't time for such considerations. I knew better and decided I would do my part to try to forge an effective Nurse-Patient relationship, even if none of them perceived it as a priority.

This bespectacled Doctor was the person leading the team responsible for saving my life. I knew if I didn't respond, he might think I wasn't cognitively intact or impaired to some degree. I had to answer all his questions so he could perform an accurate assessment and I could go home as soon as possible. I opened my eyes once again and was surprised to see several people standing motionless around the cart staring at me while others continued to remain in full motion just beyond them.

I knew this hospital was one of the largest teaching hospitals in the area, so some of those present had to be Medical Students or Residents. *"Thank God this is September, and the new Residents, if there were any in the room, have at least two month's experience. Their academic year starts in July. Would they allow first-year Residents in the Trauma Bay?"* Of course they must, but as an educator, I prided myself on not traumatizing (no pun intended) new students. Now in the role of patient, that meant I must accept that first-year Residents may provide care to me in this Trauma Bay and even possibly help save my life.

Stop worrying about who is in the room. Just cooperate, OK?

The anonymous periphery muscled its way in, and many things happened at once. The sharp poke of an IV being started in my left arm was the first thing to capture my attention. I hate having IVs started or blood drawn—I doubt anyone likes that. In the past, I was labeled a 'hard stick,' but today, I was relieved to feel the pain of that first stick quickly dissipate and observe a Nurse hang fluids. She got it on the first attempt. Good. There's something about starting an IV on the first attempt that is very vindicating for many Nurses. "Say a quick IV prayer before trying, and you'll get it," one of the 'nice' Nurses told me just after graduation. "If you can't get it after two tries, hand it off to another Nurse."

This Nurse 'got it' on the first try, but I don't think she said a prayer, was impressed with herself, or cared that much. She was simply unconsciously competent in starting IVs so the team could take over and get to the 'good stuff.' I'm sure she, too, was ready to move on to additional orders within an algorithm of care for patients who 'fell from ladders.' The energy level in the room continued to explode with the intensity that must attract Nurses and other medical professionals to work in the Emergency Department or Trauma Care settings.

IV fluids now flowing, I assessed my IV site. A quick look at the bag of fluids showed normal saline was infusing at about 100 ccs per hour via a #18 angiocath (large needle with a green hub) in the left antecubital (inner elbow) area. No erythema (redness), swelling, or discharge were noted. *Green tea…18 is an easy way to remember the color*, as I told my students many, many times.

As indicated on their ID badges, two Nurse Technicians stood on either side of me and brandished blunt bandage shears. The shears felt very cold as they grazed over my skin. Without asking permission or informing me of their intentions, my pants and shirt were quickly cut off and tossed into the biohazard container.

"My shirt? Really? That was my favorite shirt. Come on!!! Bye shirt, I hate to see you go." I watched as the comfortable go-to shirt I often wore to family events was introduced to its final resting place--the biohazard bin.

From former experience, I knew one classification of biohazardous waste was cloth or bandages that were saturated with blood. Bandages and other items with just a few drops of dried blood could be placed in a regular trash can. Come to think of it, my shirt and pants were *covered* with bloodstains, so I guess they did belong in the biohazard container. My poor clothes. May they rest in peace. "Please check the pockets," I called out over the din and then heard a voice say, "already done." I turned my attention to the voice's owner and saw it belonged to one of the Nurse Technicians inventorying my wallet, keys, a pen, and whatever else was in my pockets. I wished I had the presence of mind to give them to Ellen but knew they would be stored under lock and key for pick up later.

As I spoke, I felt the blood on my face was mostly dry, so I assumed the bleeding had slowed or stopped. My thoughts drifted to the idea of wrapping me in a blanket to protect my sister's new car upholstery. She had her old car for over ten years and worked so hard for this new shiny black model with the light grey upholstery our mom warned her might "show the dirt (or in this case, blood)." I would feel just terrible if it was ruined, especially since it's so hard, no almost impossible, to remove blood stains.

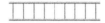

I transitioned back to reality as I felt the damp gooey stickiness of electrodes on my chest. I had shown students hundreds of times how to apply the electrodes by first helping them palpate the landmarks: "mid-clavicular lines, intercostal spaces…snow over grass, smoke over fire…" Far from being sweaty, I was cold, dry, and not at all hairy, so the Nurse tech would not have difficulty with electrode placement. I always felt sorry for the very hairy men whose chests had to be shaved using the dull single-blade disposable razors found in hospitals. When they arrived on the inpatient floor from the Emergency Room, I applied lotion to the reddened, excoriated areas that fell victim to those razors. I knew, however, the electrodes would stick to my chest very well and took comfort in that.

They placed me on the heart monitor and a number of them, including me, turned in unison to inspect the rhythm. "Sinus tachycardia, heart rate 130." *Elevated heart rate, but that's perfectly understandable given the trauma and pain.* They apparently weren't impressed by the rate or rhythm either, as their eyes quickly turned to more carefully scrutinize my body.

Please stop staring.

I am very, *very* modest about showing my body in public. I *never* go shirtless and haven't done so since elementary school when I was chubby but blissfully unaware. Lots of body shaming later, I was mortified to be lying nearly naked on a gurney with over a dozen people staring at me. I took some comfort, however, that most everything, including my man boobs, had fallen quite nicely into place in the recumbent position.

My body image was heavily influenced by growing up in a 'lookist and ageist' society. Nearly twenty years earlier, I had a severe gall bladder attack and drove myself to this same Emergency Room. Before I left the house, I showered thoroughly and even broke open a pack of new briefs and t-shirts from the previous Christmas, so I would be clean and well-dressed when the doctor saw me. Ironically, the gallstone passed on the way to the hospital, and I returned home, but still, I had made an effort to present myself as clean and tidy, as I felt that was quite simply the civilized thing to do.

There was nothing civil about my presentation on this day. I hadn't even showered, let alone put on clean underwear, and was hence wholly horrified. I knew the team wasn't looking at my body to critique it but to perform their assessment and provide life-saving care. This was no time for modesty or embarrassment. I knew any professional wouldn't be paying attention to a patient's appearance right now, so I closed my eyes and tried to go back to Bermuda while they did their work.

"BP's a little high," I heard someone call out. "Does he have a history of high blood pressure?" "No, he doesn't," I muttered softly in a feeble act of defiance against being called 'he' for the third time but then spoke more loudly. "My blood pressure is usually a bit low but must be elevated due to the pain........"

Someone bumped into my right arm again, this time much harder.

AHHHHHHHHHHHHHHHHHHHHHHHHHH
I screamed very loudly in a most guttural manner and thrust both arms outward reflexively, causing even more pain. I'm sure it echoed throughout the entire Emergency Department. I immediately regretted it and hoped the noise hadn't disturbed or frightened any other patients. *See, you're thinking about others. Perhaps there was room for a bit of civility after all.*

Then again, what else could I do but scream? Someone, I believe one of the Nurse Technicians, had attempted to move my right hand (which, according to both Nurse Erica and me, had an "obvious deformity") with no forewarning and primal instinct just took over. I lifted my left hand toward my face as more tears flowed involuntarily.

"Sir, you can't hit anybody, ok?" someone called out. Hadn't I just thought of civility? I couldn't open my eyes to see who was speaking. The pain wouldn't let me. I just called out, "I wasn't trying to hit anyone. If I moved, it was just a reflex. Please don't touch my right hand! Please! And while you're at it, please don't label me an aggressive patient. I'm a nice guy who just happens to be in a lot of pain!" No one said anything else, and I felt extraordinarily vindicated when I heard another voice chastising the first voice for touching a limb with such an 'obvious deformity.' *Be patient.* We are at a teaching hospital, and there are those present who *must be taught.* *Eyes closed…relax…back to Bermuda…*

CHAPTER 8

MAY I HAVE YOUR ATTENTION PLEASE!

There are moments in life when it is all turned inside out—what is real becomes unreal, what is unreal becomes tangible, and all your levelheaded efforts to keep a tight ontological control are rendered silly and indulgent.
Aleksandar Hemon

DESPITE UNBEARABLE PAIN, I endured several sets of hands assessing other areas of my body even before the attending Physician returned for *his* assessment. "Did he hit his head?" asked another disembodied voice. By this time, I had officially given up. Someone said. "I don't know," while another called out even louder, "does anyone know if this guy hit his head?" I opened my eyes and saw the attending, now officially identified as the bespectacled gentleman wearing a white lab coat, peering down at me and holding a penlight to assess my pupillary response.

"Oh goody. Now it's time for the good doctor to assess my cardinal fields of gaze."

I'd instructed students how to perform this skill many times in the Nursing Skills Lab. *I wonder if he will use the H pattern or the star pattern. I usually teach the star.* At just that moment, someone bumped into my right hand again, causing another jolt of excruciating pain that was worse, if even possible, than the others. I'm not sure it was the pain that pushed me over the edge, but after hearing one more round of "did he hit his head?" this Nurse had had enough.

"MAY I HAVE YOUR ATTENTION, PLEASE?" I attempted to sit up as two sets of huge hands belonging to the two male Nurse Technicians firmly held me down. "No, don't push me down. Listen to me!" They pushed me down anyway. I wasn't going anywhere but continued to yell. *"Pressured, rambling thoughts, here is your moment. Let them have it! This is all their fault."*

"My name is Dr. David Foley, and I am an Assistant Professor of Nursing with 14 years of teaching experience, even more years nursing experience, a former hospital administrator, compliance surveyor….. Will you all please listen to me? Stop calling me 'he!' Do you realize how non-therapeutic your communication is right now? Please stop referring to me in the third person!

How about *asking your patient* if he hit his head! I'm *right* here, folks, so ask ME! Now let's get it together!"

Uh oh. You just blew your cover, Dr. Foley.

Uncomfortable pause and even more awkward silence. I think I even heard a caregiver or two utter a few profane words as they conveyed their surprise. Despite the activity, everyone in Trauma Bay 1 was focused on me. I'm not sure if they listened, but they were undoubtedly staring. Some unkind thoughts about incompetence swirled in my head and almost made it to my tongue, but instead, I concluded my tirade with, "This is no way to initiate an effective therapeutic alliance with your patient! Now that I've told you who I am, I can also tell you today is Thursday, September 29th. I'm in Trauma Bay 1, and I'm here because a ladder collapsed. All the essential data elements to *prove* I'm alert and oriented times 4 and neurologically intact. To my knowledge, *I DID NOT HIT MY HEAD.* If you would have asked your patient, 'he' *WOULD HAVE TOLD YOU*!!!"

The silence that followed was long, pregnant, and desperately uncomfortable.

Brace yourself, smart aleck Nurse Foley.

The attending stared intently at me for a couple of seconds. Was he angry? Perhaps so, but it was hard for me to tell. Once he started speaking, he didn't seem mad at all but replied in a relaxed, cool manner, "Just relax, Dr. Foley. Since you *are* an Assistant Professor of Nursing with 14 years of teaching experience and even more years of nursing experience, you should know we usually assume *everyone* who falls from a ladder has a closed head injury and might not be able to respond. We'll talk to you more in a second, but right now, we need to look at your facial wound."

Oh. He wasn't unkind, just matter-of-fact. I'm sure he had heard much worse from patients during his career. At least I hadn't used profanity or directly insulted any of the team on a personal level. I've experienced the wrath of many patients, and even though I tried to filter their words as representations of their pain, injury, or illness, it's still hard to resist the temptation of letting those words take root. I hope they understood it was the pain speaking and not me, Assistant Professor of Nursing Dr. Foley.

Most of the crowd was already closely gathered around the gurney, but those who were not turned to hear my short diatribe. The realization I was lying there nearly naked, quite dirty, malodorous, body-conscious, and in excruciating pain had pushed me to the edge. So this is what that felt like: a sudden, traumatically-externalized locus of control. As I often told students, a clinical and rather technical way of saying you have lost your independence and ability to care for yourself.

I think that's what finally did it.

I closed my eyes and started to weep from a special, private place I had only entered a few times before in my life, like the times when one of my loved ones died. I didn't weep because I was transported back to nursing school and felt like the student Nurse whose feelings were hurt by an angry doctor or the unbearable pain. I also didn't weep because I had just heard someone call for a plastic Surgeon whispering, "This guy has a nasty through and through facial laceration." I cried solely because I knew too much about what was happening to me and had just tasted reality.

As a Nurse, I knew what lay ahead: a long, painful recovery from these severe injuries as well as the anticipated depression, despair, emotional upheaval, and lifestyle change. Several questions formed a tempest in my mind in no particular order: what about my elderly parents? I considered myself to be an integral part of their support system. I invite them to dinner frequently and, more importantly, take my mom out to lunch and shopping on Saturdays. She appreciates getting out of the house. How could I disappoint her? What will happen to them?

Who will care for my family of three cats? I live alone and have grown to appreciate the value their simple, unconditional love brings to my life. I am tempted to say I spoil them, but it's more accurate to say we spoil *each other*. They wait for me by the front door each evening, wanting only food and love. They give so much in return I almost feel selfish receiving it. Although they don't require a good deal of maintenance, they need food and water, daily litter box scooping, and weekly litter box changes. It would be a long time until I could do those tasks again, but I'm sure they would still love me even if someone else fed them, changed their water, scooped, or changed the litter.

"Am I less of a man for admitting I like cats so much?"

Reality intruded into my thoughts and screamed: *"Wake up! You're probably going to have to stay in the hospital for a while, but let's hope you don't have to go to rehab. You broke both arms but probably didn't break any bones in your legs. That helps. You just have to go home. There's so much to do…you can find ways to adapt somehow."*

What about the publications and correspondence on my computer's desktop? As a new doctoral graduate, technically a 'post doc,' I had much to address. The first post doc year is essential: establish a writing and research agenda, network, perform guest lectures, attend conferences and perhaps even get some grant funding. Working at a state-supported school with a teaching focus, I still hoped to do research and obtain a highly sought-after grant. What about my committee work? It was progressing so well. We were getting very close to completing our all-faculty proposal to realign the School's theoretical framework. No small task given all the opinions in the room, but we were making progress, nonetheless.

My class! I'm currently teaching Psychiatric-Mental Health Nursing, the essential elements of which were the source of my clinical interests: psycho-social assessment, stress, adaptation, and therapeutic communication. Only four weeks into the course, we were ready to discuss psychotic disorders, most notably Schizophrenia. I had just spent two weeks discussing the topic of mental status evaluation. I was so intrigued by the thought of bringing those concepts to life through a robust, interactive classroom discussion involving a case study I had just authored.

During the four years I had taught the course, we progressed from having no students identify psychiatric-mental health nursing as their specialty of choice to having at least 3-4 from each graduating class actively seek employment within the discipline. In fact, at the time of this accident, two former students had been accepted into graduate school to become Nurse Practitioners. I took pride in that fact and must admit I was protective—no, a bit territorial—about the course. It would be quite narcissistic to think no one but me could teach the class. That was not the case. I just really enjoyed teaching it and wanted the students to connect with the discipline and learn as much as possible.

In addition, my work ethic was a big part of my identity, and a protracted absence would be highly distressing. Be prompt, show up for work, and work hard. It was a formula that served me so well in the past, even during challenging times like working full-time and attending nursing school, graduate school, or doctoral studies. I knew I would have to be 'out sick,' and that bothered me terribly.

Did he hit his head indeed? The basic fact was, as a Nurse, I just knew too much about the world of healthcare, nursing, traumatic injury, and recovery, and I was utterly overwhelmed. I was the one who always took care of others, but this time I was the patient and wondered who would care for me and those I loved. That wondering made me very scared, especially as I lay there cold, in extreme pain, and trembling uncontrollably.

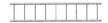

There was a momentary lull in activity as the team strategized and discussed their plans for my care. During this time, I basked in a few minutes of self-indulged pity then regained my composure. I also reaffirmed my vow to take in every sight, sound, feeling, sensation, and spoken word of this experience, vowing to share everything with students. If I couldn't be there to teach my course, then at least I would gather plenty of stories to share with them. What a tremendous pedagogical strategy: use all of this as a personal story…

I felt a sensation near my left arm and opened my eyes to see Nurse Vivian walking away. She must have slipped me some pain medication through my IV port while I was deep in thought because I felt a strange floating sensation, not like the sensation of falling asleep, but the haze induced by a narcotic. I've always had a very low tolerance for pain medications, meaning any prescription for narcotics usually went unfilled. Acetaminophen was generally more than sufficient to address my pain needs, and so whatever she gave felt very powerful. My care team decided to bring out the big guns, especially after my rant. I never determined what medication it was, but it was overwhelming. Maybe if my arm hadn't been bumped twice, I wouldn't have needed it so much…

I was floating, and the pain seemed much farther away. *Very sneaky but effective, Nurse Vivian.* Still deeply in thought, I hoped I was medicated because of my pain and not simply to silence a patient who was being too vocal.

Blissful sleep….

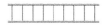

Someone was moving the cart, resulting in a quick trip back to reality. I was disoriented for just a moment but quickly reclaimed my awareness. I was informed I was going to X-ray, but not to worry. I would be transported right on this very cart. "David, you need to go to X-ray," the attending said with assured confidence. It's obvious your right wrist is broken, but we need to make sure nothing else is broken in your right arm."

"My left arm is broken too. It's very weak. I think my left wrist and elbow are broken," I said. *"Please," I thought, "I was just starting to feel comfortable. Can't I just lay here a while longer and go to X-ray later?"*

"No, I doubt your left arm is broken," he said. "You just lay back, relax as best you can, and let us do the diagnosing. It looks like your left arm is OK to me, but I will order X-rays if it makes you happy." *Make me happy? At this point, the only thing that would make me happy today is to get out of this hospital and not have the pleasure of seeing you again, Doctor.*

He turned to one of the Residents and said, "I sure hope he didn't hit his head."

The 'he' and the 'head' again. Just because I make a statement that there might be something wrong with a part of my body that means I may have a head injury? Didn't they hear anything I said earlier?

He, he, he…

A male Transporter was at the head of the gurney and began to push it out of Trauma Bay 1. I was so glad I didn't have to transfer to another cart and move from my semi-comfortable position. All I had to do was simply lay in one place and be mindful to keep my hands perfectly still. I tried to place them on my chest, but they hurt too much. "Are the side rails locked?" I asked, wanting to avoid tumbling onto the floor. *Wouldn't that be terrible? A patient fall from a cart while leaving the Trauma Bay? Imagine that Root Cause Analysis…*

No one answered me.

The trip to Radiology was safe, smooth, and efficient. The X-ray technician was as gentle as she could be in positioning my hand and arms for each of the images. No matter how carefully she moved, however, I became insane from the pain associated with each new repositioning and asked her to *please* call for some medication. "I wonder if it's time for pain medication, even a sledgehammer," I joked. "Please, I really need something. I just can't take it anymore. Please." She excused herself momentarily to communicate my request. After she completed the series of X-rays, she informed me I would wait in the hallway until it was time for the CT Scan of my head. She apologetically explained that other patients also needed a CT Scan, and they would see me as soon as possible. *I guess there are people in worse shape than you, Nurse Foley. Good sign, but a CT Scan? The head again. Well, he had to order that, didn't he?* The hallway was quite busy, and I was extraordinarily self-conscious, praying the pain medication would arrive soon.

Just then, a silver-haired male Nurse appeared. No surprise, as many men self-select into nursing's critical-care or technical disciplines. So many thoughts came to mind based on my doctoral research: men choosing the most socially acceptable roles within a female-dominated profession, critical care, crisis, rescuer, leader, equipment-based... A sardonic view of men in nursing, but I suppose it's at least partially true.

I smiled weakly and pleasantly greeted him, but he offered only a terse "hello" with no eye contact, a flat affect, and a monotone voice. *"Good thing you self-selected into Emergency or Trauma Medicine. Nursing's 'softer' disciplines like Obstetrics, Pediatrics, and Psychiatry wouldn't want you and your flat affect. Say something. Smile at least..."*

He walked deeper into the room and sharply asked the Radiology Technician, "Is that him?" Mind you, he didn't ask *me* who was laying right there and happened to be the 'him' in the equation. Once I was identified by proxy, the silver-haired male Nurse quickly grabbed the IV tubing, found a port, attached the syringe, and blasted a substance into my bloodstream. Administration time? About two seconds.

As he tossed the syringe into the sharps container, he turned to me, a Nurse Educator and a huge proponent for men in nursing, and said, "consider that a special delivery. It might make you feel funny for a while" and turned to chat with the congenial X-ray technician.

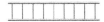

Quick interlude, sir...

OK really?

Unknown silver-haired male Nurse, you just failed your nursing skills check. I regret to inform you I must send you back to the Nursing Skills Lab to remediate for the following reasons:

- Did you utilize two unique identifiers like full name and date of birth to make sure the 'him' was me? NO
- Did you verify my drug allergies? NO
- Did you inform me what you were going to do? NO
- Did you identify the name of the medication you were administering? NO
- Did you scrub the IV port before administering the medication to minimize the risk of infection? NO
- Did you don gloves before administering? NO
- Did you push the medication slowly over...I don't know... at least 2 minutes to minimize dizziness or nausea? NO

*You **FLUNKED**, and I am not giving you a pass just for trying. Back to the lab you go, and don't' come back until you know what you're doing! You might really hurt someone...*

I would never say that to a student, but in this case, his gross incompetence as a practicing Nurse made the words seem appropriate.

End interlude and back to reality. But really, sir…we need to talk about your nursing practice sometime…

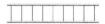

Almost immediately, I became unbelievably dizzy, felt a strange fluttering in my heart, and had difficulty breathing while the room began to dance within my field of vision. I clawed the cart's sheet with my left in an attempt to grab onto *something*. I couldn't breathe and was terrified—fear associated with air hunger. The whole experience lasted about five minutes and was just horrible.

Had I known, I would have toughed it out and asked Nurse Vivian for pain medication when I got back to the Trauma Bay. I didn't know her very well yet, but I bet she at least scrubbed the port before she gave me pain medication. Inept, insensitive, self-selecting critical care silver-haired Nurse, will you take your medication back and let me start over? Nurse Vivian would have passed *her* skill check.

This male RN, who never did introduce himself, stood and talked with the X-ray technician just a few feet from me while I endured the episode of irregular heartbeats and difficulty breathing. During the highly unnerving experience, he glanced over once or twice, but I assume he interpreted my quietness as though I was experiencing the medication's therapeutic benefits.

He turned abruptly and left the room and my life, but not my memory.

No, unknown male Nurse. You and your unsafe nursing practice will reside in my memory for a very long time, but at least I can use you as an example of deplorable nursing practice. Thank you for that, at least.

I still had to endure the CT scan of the head, but by that point, my body had adjusted to the pain medication, and I was feeling a bit more comfortable. The test, as it turned out, wasn't so bad. I had always imagined I would be terrified if I had to go into the machine, but since the scan involved only my head, it was over in just a few noisy minutes. The transport back to Trauma Bay 1 was tolerable, thanks to my 'special delivery,' so I greeted Nurse Vivian as pleasantly as circumstances would allow and settled in for the next round of the unknown.

CHAPTER 9

FIGURE IT OUT, PLEASE!

Apprehension, uncertainty, waiting, expectation, fear of surprise, do a patient more harm than any exertion. Remember he is face to face with his enemy all the time.
Florence Nightingale

SINCE IT WAS relatively apparent my injuries were not life-threatening, the crowd in the room had dispersed and moved on to their next challenge. That left only Nurse Vivian, a first-year medical student named Allan, and two Residents, all of whom are listed in my perceived order of their importance. Nurse Vivian was first on the list because she spoke directly to me and seemed to be in charge. I wasn't sure about Allan. He was quietly polite but made direct eye contact and seemed bright and attentive. Allan's body language conveyed he was in Trauma Bay 1 for the long haul, and I found comfort in that.

I also ranked the Residents last because they never really spoke to me, and I had no idea why they were there. I got the distinct impression they were bored with the scene in Trauma Bay 1 and wanted to see some 'real action.' With this hospital's designation as a clinical teaching site, it was readily apparent a number of those in the initial larger crowd were students, there to learn as much as they possibly could. I almost sensed their disappointment as they left, realizing there wasn't anything exciting with my case that could capture their attention for very long. Based on their body language, the Residents felt the same way.

Sorry to disappoint you, folks!

Their lack of interest, though, made me surmise the outcome wasn't as bleak as my mind had imagined. Once the attending and entourage left to see the next case, Nurse Vivian completely took over. There was something very comforting in the fact that a Nurse had assumed control.

Take us there, Spartacus!

I witnessed her effortlessly bring to life many of the concepts I discussed with students: organization, advocacy, caring, therapeutic communication, and technical prowess. She helped the Residents prioritize my care and treatment. "OK, gentlemen, let's take a look at these

X-rays. We need to know what's going on with both of his arms." Both of my arms? Maybe Nurse Vivian believed me when I said there was something wrong with my left arm!

I drifted off to sleep for a few minutes, but the strong cadence of her voice roused me as she said to the Orthopedic and Plastic Surgery Residents, "no, you are *not* working on his face and arms at the same time. Figure it out, please." What was going on? Apparently, the Orthopedic and Plastic Surgery Residents had arrived simultaneously and wanted to set my right arm and suture my face simultaneously. As they continued to argue, she said once again, "If you can't figure it out, I will get the attending," after which the Plastic Surgery Residents impatiently agreed they could wait a few minutes.

"Well played, Miss Vivian," I whispered to myself. She also directed Allan, now hovering in the back of the room, to stand next to me "…so you can talk to this patient and learn something." When he didn't react, she said, "there's no need to be shy. Just observe and ask him how he is doing from time to time, that's all. It's important for patients just to know someone is here for them." Allan patted me on my shoulder in a most caring and not at all patronizing manner. "Please let me know if you need anything. I'm a medical student, but I can help too."

Oh, Miss Vivian, you are a Nurse among Nurses. Look what you just did. You taught a young medical student the basics of therapeutic communication…mindfulness, eye contact, therapeutic touch…Now, will you please speak to

Mr. Silver-haired 'special delivery Nurse?' He needs your consultative services at once!

Vivian then stopped to speak directly to me. "David, we have a short break in the action before they start working on your arms and face. Is there anyone in the waiting room you would like us to notify?"

MY SISTER!!!

"Yes, my sister Ellen is in the Waiting Room. Can you bring her back, please? I'm sure it would make her *(and me)* feel better to step in." I had no idea how much time had elapsed, but it seemed like so long since I had seen her. I wonder if she was sitting out there alone. If she was, I'm sure she was frightened. Despite my injuries, I felt for her. I just hoped I looked a little more presentable than the last time she saw me..."Ok," Vivian replied, "just for a minute, though." "Do I look OK?" I asked her. "Good idea," she replied and quickly grabbed a washcloth and cleaned my face. Its coolness felt wonderful, but I noted she avoided the area around my nose and upper lip. "That's the best I can do for now. Let me go get her before they get started." She looked at the two Residents and said, "Get set up for his right arm. You will need the hand trap to immobilize. You're going to sedate him, right? Set up, but don't start until I return." With that, she turned on her heel and quickly disappeared.

When she left, I turned my attention to Allan, who was now second on my list of favorite Trauma Bay 1 caregivers. He looked so young, possibly in his early twenties. I asked him how far along he was in medical school, and he said "first year." He seemed uneasy and a bit awkward. I thanked him for standing with me, and from that moment until I left Trauma Bay 1, he occasionally placed his hand on my shoulder said, "how are you doing, David? Let us know if you need anything or have any questions. We're here for you."

"Thank you, that means a lot."

Interdisciplinary education in action. The University just built a 40 million dollar building so doctors and Nurses can learn together, and now here we are. In different circumstances, I would have liked to place a nursing student with him to experience this together. Better yet, it would be fascinating to have both write and share reflective journals so they could compare and contrast each other's impressions of the experience...

Just then, the attending Physician abruptly returned and told the Residents my right arm had a clean fracture at the ulna and radius but was only severely bruised at the right elbow. The wrist (ulna and radial fractures) needed to be reset, or at least I think that's what he said. "What about my left arm? It's broken too," I interrupted. "No," he said, "your left arm is *not*" broken. "Let me be the doctor here, Dr. Foley," followed by nervous laughter from the Residents. "Doctor, I'm *sorry*...but my left arm *is* broken. I have generalized weakness in my left elbow and sharp pain upon movement in my left wrist. I think it's broken—or at least sprained—in both places. Please, doctor," I continued calmly, "listen to the patient. They *know their own bodies*," speaking to him, but also looked pleadingly from Resident to Resident.

What was taking Nurse Vivian so long?

I knew my words would make him angry, but they sounded good anyway. I had advocated for patients so many times during my career, but never for myself, or at least not like this. What choice did I have? Be meekly submissive and leave my left arm untreated just to avoid his wrath? I never fully understood why he engaged in a battle of wills with me over my left arm, but he did. *Even more concerning, what about the patients who didn't understand the concept of power dynamics in the Patient-Caregiver relationship and unquestioningly accepted his direction?* The worst that could happen in my case was he would become angry, but no, that's not the worst that could happen. The worst that could happen was my left arm *was* broken. Two broken arms, a facial injury, loss of independence, and some unsafe practice was getting close to the 'worst that could happen' category, and quite honestly, I didn't care if the good doctor was angry or not.

He did appear quite perturbed, but before he could speak, Nurse Vivian returned with Ellen. I realized Nurse Vivian probably took some time to update her about my care and provide her with a dose of comfort and reassurance. She brought her into Trauma Bay 1 and then disappeared out of view. Ellen stood quietly for a few moments and just looked at me, unsure what to do. At the same time, I heard Nurse Vivian's voice as she asked the team about my X-rays and inquired about my left arm. The Residents had looked at the X-rays and determined I *did* have an avulsion fracture in my left elbow and a fracture of the Triquetral bone of the left wrist. Was I satisfied? No, considering both of my arms required attention, but I must admit I was just a little bit pleased about being right.

OK, admit it, you feel happy and vindicated. What would the attending's reaction be?

"David, how are you?" my sister asked, and I could tell she had been crying. The long wait had not been kind to her. "I'm going to be OK," I assured her. "Did they give you my phone, wallet, and keys?" She assured me she had them in her purse. "Good. Get my phone and call my work. Dial this number. Go." Without thinking, she retrieved my phone—complete with a smear of dried blood—dialed the number, and put the phone to my ear. Thankfully someone answered, a rare occurrence in the School of Nursing during busy afternoon hours, and I asked the staff member to please bring the Associate Dean to the phone—it was an emergency…in the hospital…. hurt… She transferred the call, and I got her voice mail.

"Are you kidding me? Call again, please." A quick redial and the Associate Dean herself answered apologetically. I told her where I was and what had happened. "I'm not technically due in until Monday, but I wanted you to know now because you'll need to make arrangements for coverage."

Me, the employee who never, ever misses work, is now calling in four days in advance for my Monday classes. There was a relatively long moment of silence while she processed. This must be serious. "We're coming over there now," she interrupted me.

"We?"

"Yes, I'll see who's available, and we'll be right over."

"Oh no, that's OK, my sister's here, and I'm sure some of my family will be on their way over too." Although I appreciated the gesture, I didn't want any of my work colleagues to see me in this condition. "Are you sure?" she asked? "Yes," I was sure, but I wanted to tell them, even as I lay in Trauma Bay 1, not to expect me at work anytime soon and so they could make plans for coverage. Always the administrator and pragmatist, I suppose I wanted to update her but didn't expect them to come over and sit with me. The Associate Dean said, "Forget about that now. We'll take care of the details later. Focus on *you.*"

No argument from me. I will gladly take you up on that.

I caught the eye of the attending staring at me intently and slowly shaking his head. His look said, *"Are you kidding me?"* but at the same time, I think he understood. Knowing how difficult it would be to find coverage, I felt I needed to let the School know as soon as possible, and I returned his gaze with equal intensity.

At least he knows now that you really are an Assistant Professor of Nursing…

I not only begged but *begged* my sister not to call my elderly parents. It was Thursday afternoon, and my mom's weekly visit with me wasn't until Saturday morning, so I had the luxury of at least 24 hours before I had to tell them and hoped I would be a bit more presentable by then. I couldn't imagine how upset they would be when they learned of the accident. "Do you want me to tell anyone else?" "Absolutely not, "I replied, "no one."

"Time to go, hon," Nurse Vivian told my sister and whisked her back into the waiting room. "Love you," I called out after my sister, who turned, waved, and offered a feeble smile. I wished I had taken more time to ask her how she was doing rather than worry about my job. Still, I knew if she could survive the happenings of this terrible afternoon, she could manage a few more hours waiting in an inner-city emergency department's waiting room.

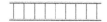

"Let's get to work, David," Nurse Vivian told me confidently upon her return. Along with the two still-nameless Residents, she turned to caucus with the attending, leaving only Allan, who never once moved from his position at the head of the exam table. We all listened carefully while the attending spoke directly to me. "We need to fix the gross deformity in your right arm. To do that, we're going to give you medicine to put you in a twilight state. If there's any good news in this, your right arm is badly bruised but not broken anywhere else, and there's no evidence of head trauma.

"Wow, the CT scan results came in fast," I offered, but no one paid attention.

"While you're sleeping, they're also going to put a temporary splint on your left arm. It's also broken at the wrist and has an avulsion fracture at the elbow, but there's nothing to set. We will let the Orthopedic attending decide whether to cast it or not." He made direct eye contact with me, and a few tears involuntarily splashed from each eye.

There's no victory in self-diagnosing my left arm, doctor. How about a just bit of empathy? How would I cope with two broken arms? How could I work, care for my loved ones...just live? I wanted to tell him that but kept the comments to myself.

Nurse Vivian placed a carbon dioxide monitor in my nostrils and asked the Residents, who I learned were first-year Orthopedic Residents, to wait until she had a set of vitals before administering the sedative. *I recalled 'pre-induction' vitals must be taken before sedation is administered from previous experience with compliance surveys...*

A Resident came bursting in with what looked like an IV pole from which small net-like devices were hanging in a row. Another eager Resident supported my right elbow and forearm while the other guided my hand to insert my thumb and four fingers into their respective net-like traps. It turned out once my fingers were slipped into these net-like traps, my arm could be suspended to assist with re-aligning the broken bones through gravity and then manual manipulation.

"Doctor, should you be doing that before I am sedated? Please don't let GOOOOOOOOOOOOOOO," I screamed as he unexpectedly pulled back and let my arm swing freely before any medication was given. My pain rating had settled into a reasonably comfortable "3" but immediately became unimaginable. I screamed another primal scream that sent the attending's pen flying as he dashed to the bedside, uttering some very colorful language. He personally provided support to my arm and actually apologized after telling the Resident to step back. "Give it *now*," he ordered, and Nurse Vivian, apparently satisfied that all pre-anesthesia requirements had been met, did so without speaking.

Please don't leave the bedside again, Nurse Vivian. I need you here.

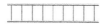

I awoke to find my right arm tightly bound in a temporary cast consisting of a plastic splint covered by cotton batting and several ace wraps. I knew that because I asked for details as soon as the haze began to lift. My left arm was also splinted and similarly wrapped. I was surprised how lucid I was, especially given I had just received sedation but recalled the medication was very short-acting. A person I didn't recognize said quite apologetically, "We're from the Plastics Hand Service and will be taking care of your right wrist. We also wrapped your left arm just to be cautious. You will see the Orthopedic attending soon, and he will decide if your left arm needs to be casted or not. Until then, you will have very little use of either of your arms and hands. I'm sorry. We don't want any of your fractures to get any worse until you are seen." I tried to tell him both of the wraps seemed unreasonably tight, but he disappeared out of my small field of vision, and I never saw him again.

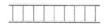

Just a few minutes later, a frightfully young-looking woman appeared in Trauma Bay 1. She was wearing a colorful jean jacket, short pleated jean skirt over black tights, patent leather shoes, a ponytail, and was carrying a small backpack over her shoulder. I thought maybe she was a lost high school student on a field trip, but she locked eyes with me and said very pleasantly, "Hello, I'm Rachel, the Senior Plastic Surgery Resident, and I'm going to be putting your face back together."

WHAT?????? You've got to be kidding!!!!!

She calmly and pleasantly continued. "It looks like you have a 'through and through lip lac (laceration)' that needs immediate attention. Let me see." Rubber gloves in place, Dr. Rachel summoned over the Residents and said, "See," gently tapping her petite index finger through the hole to touch my upper gum. My wide eyes must have conveyed a strong sense of concern because she asked, "Has anyone talked with you about this yet?"

"Uh uh," I shook my head slightly. "They have not. How bad is it? Fixable?"

"Of course," she said. "We can fix this" as she dragged over a small step stool with her foot, climbed atop it, and firmly established herself at the head of the cart. It seemed so odd to have someone standing over me and upside down in my field of vision, especially as the last whispers of the short-acting anesthesia were subsiding. She continued authoritatively, "Let's see inside. Hmmm....Oh." Motioning two newly-arrived plastic surgery Residents to Trauma Bay 1, she quietly pointed out that somehow my upper lip must have caught something during the fall, violently stretching my lip upward. The force ultimately resulted in about 4" of my upper gum being traumatically severed, all the way to the bone capsule.

I had not noticed the pain in my mouth until Dr. Rachel began her examination. Tears reflexively streamed down my face while I made direct eye contact with her upside-down visage. "Do you want him asleep for this?" Nurse Vivian asked. Thanks for asking, Nurse Vivian. I was just thinking the same thing. *Please put me back to sleep. The sedation was just beautiful.*

"No, we'll just do local," Dr. Rachel replied.

Darn!

Allan, still keeping faithful watch near my head, placed his hand firmly on my shoulders and said, "I bet this is going to really hurt David. If you want to grab my hand, go for it. Just know I'm here for you, ok, and whatever you do, please don't move."

Good man! I might just take you up on your offer, and no, I won't move.

The Residents administered the local anesthetic via several injections, many of which appeared to penetrate almost to the bone. I groaned, and tears flowed freely. I knew I couldn't move, but on at least two occasions, it took every ounce of my being not to knock their hands out of the way…but then again, my hands were wrapped and completely useless. Since the accident, the pain in my right arm overrode every other sensation in my body, including this four-inch tear in my gum tissue and 'through and through lip lac,' Now that my mouth was front and center, I was back in misery's camp and looking for an escape route.

Nurse Vivian, I felt so comfortable when you were here. Where do you go?

Dr. Rachel re-positioned herself on the stool that gave her the needed height to view the surgical site properly. "Doctor, before you get started, I'd like to make a deal with you. I don't care what you do, but please don't make me any uglier than I was before the accident, ok?"

"Oh, come on now," she laughed and stared at me with eyes that were now shielded by a faceguard. Some genuine, though nervous, laughter flowed throughout Trauma Bay 1 but quickly dissipated as Dr. Rachel set to work.

After about 45 minutes of suturing, tugging, and pulling (my mouth required many, many stitches to repair several different layers of tissue), my upper lip was swollen to approximately three times its normal size. The Attending stopped by and asked, "Did you lose any teeth?" "None," I replied, feeling very thankful. He watched for a few anxious seconds while I ran my tongue over my upper and lower front teeth. They felt intact and smooth. I shook my head silently.

"None? Let me see," he asked skeptically and donned a rubber glove. After close inspection, he was quite genuine when he asserted, "you are fortunate, sir! I thought we were going to have to consult the Oral-Maxillofacial Service, but I'm glad we don't have to." As he reached the charting station, I heard him say to Nurse Vivian, "how did he get a huge upper lip lac and not break any teeth? Lucky guy."

God was watching over me, Doctor.

Nurse Vivian gave me some additional pain medication using perfect technique and, in doing so, successfully passed *her* imaginary skill check. *Nicely done, Nurse Vivian.*

And with that, I fell into a deep sleep.

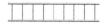

When I woke up, Dr. Rachel and her Residents, faithful Allan, and even Nurse Vivian all seemed to have disappeared. Arms casted and laceration repaired, I laid there alone with only an intense, aching pain to keep me company.

Oh no. I realized I had to urinate—very badly.

I had been receiving IV fluids at 100 ccs/hr, and it had been hours since I went. I looked around the room and saw no one, but I focused on the charting station and saw the Attending. I quietly called out my need, and he silently stepped out into the hallway. He returned with a male Nurse Technician in tow, who offered me a urinal, suggesting it would be easier to 'go' right there in the cart.

Nice try, but absolutely no way, sir.

"I can stand if you can help me walk to the commode." After the attending silently nodded his approval, the Nursing Assistant lowered the cart and side rail. "I'm going to sit up very slowly and sit at the side of the bed for a minute," I offered, "so I can give myself time to adjust to the postural change."

Are either of you impressed? I doubt it.

I slowly stood while he positioned himself directly in front of me with his arms firmly but gently planted on my shoulders. I walked very deliberately, all the while trying to figure out how I would perform the act once I arrived.

From the elbow to the tips of my fingers, my right arm was placed in a metal splint and then wrapped with a generous amount of padding, gauze, and ace wrap that made any movement of my fingers impossible. I couldn't even move my fingertips but then realized that was the point of immobilization. *But not even my fingertips?*

The fingertips on my left arm *were* exposed, allowing me to make a 'C' with my thumb and index finger, and I knew that would be just enough to snag my briefs and pull them down just enough to urinate. Of course, any movement was painful, but I endured it to avoid the 'indignity of having someone help me perform a very basic body function laying on a cart in public view. I had helped patients do that many times and thought nothing of it, but I just couldn't do that. Not now.

"Can I try going by myself?" I asked as a steel toilet amazingly swung out of the cabinet right in front of me. He said, "You better let me help you, sir," but I ignored him and urinated on my own. Why was this so traumatic for me? I had a brief flash of the work of Orem, who indicated Nurses care by being 'compensatory' only to the degree needed to address a deficit, whether an essential, ordinary task or something more life-sustaining. In this case, the Nursing Assistant was 'partially compensatory' since I could stand and urinate but needed set-up and stand-by assistance. I tried to share my thoughts with him, but he only stared at me blankly.

How many times had I calmly and cheerfully told patients, "it's no big deal...I know this is very hard for you, but trust me, we do this all the time, so please don't be embarrassed." It was extraordinary to experience someone helping me with a private act, along with the realization my aging, flawed body was nothing novel or unique. To the Nurse Technician, helping me was no big deal either. Nevertheless, I resolved I wasn't one of 'those patients'; this was *me,* and draped in denial, I was determined to overcome as quickly as possible.

Immediately following my toileting victory, the activity level picked up once again. The Attending and Nurse Vivian both reappeared, this time apparently with a single, unified purpose. "Are you ready for admission to the Trauma Unit?" he asked? "Do you have anyone in the waiting room? You'll be going up as soon as the Nurse calls report."

"Can't I go home?" I politely but abruptly asked him. "I have people who can help me, and I am worried about my cats. I'll be ok." He looked at me for a few seconds while Nurse Vivian frowned and crossed her arms. Maybe what happened next was the dramatic climax of our long, protracted unspoken battle of wills or just a bit of anger by a weary Physician nearing the end of a long shift, but he quickly grabbed a chair, sat down on it backward, and made direct eye contact with me. "No, Dr. Foley, you can't go home tonight. You can't feed yourself, you can't get up by yourself, and most importantly, you might not be able to go to the bathroom by yourself! You can sign yourself out AMA, but you know better! If you do that, you may be responsible for the entire bill. Now let us help you and just relax. You'll be going upstairs shortly. It's time for you to be the patient in this equation."

Really? Had I been *that* difficult so far or just been a rare patient who dared to speak up? I sighed, nodded my assent, and just looked away. After a moment, he got up and moved back into position with the desk acting as a protective barrier between the two of us...well... four of us if you counted our egos.

OK, Nurse Foley, lay down your arms and surrender.

He left without saying a word. I hoped he knew how grateful I was for his role as the team leader who coordinated my care during a time of crisis. Nonetheless, I hoped he also remembered to heavily scrutinize the content on 'therapeutic communication' in the nearest textbook as soon as possible.

Weary smile...

Nurse Vivian was next at bat. She had called report to the inpatient Trauma Unit, but since my bed wasn't ready, I must first be moved to a holding area in the Emergency Department so Trauma Bay 1 could be cleaned for the next case.

I hope it doesn't have to be used for a very long time, but I knew better.

Shortly after that, transport arrived, and Nurse Vivian, along with her spectacular technical acumen, marvelous communication skills, and propensity for patient advocacy, disappeared. *Bye, Nurse Vivian. You were amazing and left a great impression on me. Thank you for being an example of what a Nurse should be. Many current and future students will hear about you and the magnificence of your nursing practice. I wondered if any of the other Nurses I would encounter could possibly match your greatness.*

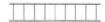

Two young and very enthusiastic Nurses greeted me in the Emergency Department's holding area. "You'll be going up to the Trauma Unit in about an hour or so," one of them said pleasantly. Trying to make conversation, I asked them about where they were in their nursing educations. They looked at me a bit quizzically but conveyed they had both completed Bachelor of Science in Nursing Programs but had not yet thought about pursuing graduate studies. After I encouraged them to do so, they seemed genuinely interested, especially when I told them never to forget to integrate the *art* of nursing into their valuable work in the Emergency Department. You know….more than just technical skills… caring… cultural competence…therapeutic communication…

After a few more pleasantries, I realized I had to urinate again. Darn those IV fluids. I asked the Nurse if the fluids could be discontinued. I promised her I would drink juice, water, whatever, and wouldn't have to pee so often if I didn't have 100cc of fluids pumped into me each hour. She smiled, made eye contact, and explained no, I could not have the fluids discontinued just yet. I had received some potent pain medication, and the fluids would help 'flush out' the narcotics and any byproducts of tissue damaged by the trauma. It was simply 'way too early' to discontinue the fluids.

Yuk.

I waited for them to leave me alone and then quickly formulated a plan.

I knew Nurse Vivian had given me one additional dose of one of those very powerful pain medications right before I left Trauma Bay, and I was definitely feeling its effects. Did I report this and ask for a urinal? Of course not. If I was reluctant to urinate in the presence of a male Nursing Assistant, how would I feel about doing so in front of these two young female Nurses?

I sat up and used my nose and the tips of any exposed finger to activate the controls to elevate the head of the bed and somehow released the side rail. I swung my legs over and used my core muscles to turn and sit at the side of the bed and then paused. *Avoid sudden postural changes, please. Let your legs dangle a while so your body can acclimate, and you won't feel dizzy when you stand.* Luckily, the IV pole was on my side of the bed, so I didn't have to worry about not having enough tubing to reach the toilet. As I stood, I extended my arms, hooked the IV pump with my left elbow, and moved slowly forward.

The pain was excruciating. I felt my heart beating in my hands, elbows, forearms, legs, and many other parts of my body. I wondered what my blood pressure might be. It was slightly elevated in the Emergency Department on arrival, but I attributed that to the accident and the pain. My feet felt so cold, and I realized I wasn't wearing any socks. I needed to ask for some hospital-issued non-skid footwear, those socks with the rubber tread to prevent falls. Not very fashion-forward, but they promote safety and warmth. I just hated the sensation of the cold tile on my feet, but there was no turning back. I traversed the 5 feet with as much dignity as I could muster and used my foot to ease the bathroom's door open.

Standing in front of the commode, I slowly and carefully used my newly discovered thumb and index "C formation" method to pull my gown aside and pull down my briefs just enough to urinate what must have seemed like half a liter. Mission completed, I felt so much better.

I turned around to see one of my Nurses standing at the door to the restroom. Uh oh. She politely—and appropriately—offered educational points about asking for help before getting out of bed and the importance of preventing falls, talking even as I was slowly walking back to the safety and comfort of the bed. Of course, I knew asking for assistance was a requirement for a patient in my condition in the Emergency Department; after all, I was a *nursing instructor! Of all people, I should understand and…well….be ashamed of myself!*

"I'm sorry," I won't do it again. I just didn't want to bother you. After a few more polite rebukes, the Nurse informed me it was time to go. My sister would meet me on the unit. *Ellen! Was she still here? Oh, I hope she had called someone to sit with her.*

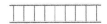

True to her word, my Nurse slowly and deliberately moved my bed out of the treatment room, down the hall, and into an elevator. As opposed to my initial arrival at the Emergency Department earlier in the day, I was too tired to look around and take in any sights and sounds. I just stared up at the ceiling, watching the lights move past until I started to feel nauseous. I hadn't eaten anything since early that morning, and I supposed that didn't help. I closed my eyes and focused on deep breathing. I heard other people conversing on the elevator, but I didn't even open my eyes this time. In fact, I didn't open them until the bed slid to a halt in my room on 5 West, the Inpatient Trauma Unit.

I was utterly exhausted, badly shaken, and ready for some real sleep. My admitting Nurse Tina arrived and pleasantly introduced herself. She would need to do an admission assessment, but since we had "all night together," she would complete it later after we both settled in.

"Oh, that's fine. I really need some rest," I told her. "Can you please find my sister and send her in?" "Of course," Nurse Tina replied, and within five minutes,

Ellen appeared at my bedside. She sat down and just stared at me. There was no more blood to see, and the initial shock of the accident was behind us. She was, however, confronted with the new sights of my grossly swollen face and both of my arms casted and prominently displayed on pillows. She looked tired and was involuntarily tearful. I told her to go home. I would be fine, and she could come and see me in the morning.

"Don't forget, I'm a Nurse, and I can handle myself in here. Just don't tell mom and dad yet but go check on the cats." A few 'I 'love yous' and some tears mixed with laughter, and she was gone. Yes, my dear sister, now I *know* you could have been a Nurse after all. Thank you for facing this day with me. Although I would always be willing, I hope never to have to do the same for you.

CHAPTER 10

HEAVENLY FIGURES

When one teaches, two learn.
Robert A. Heinlein

CLOSED MY EYES and fell into a blissfully deep, narcotics-induced sleep. I don't think Nurse Tina ever came back to do my admission. She probably completed it without my involvement and just used the information in my chart, but I didn't care. I needed the sleep, and she accommodated me.

Some hushed, whispered conversation and restrained laughter woke me. I half-opened my eyes to see several shadowy figures, most of whom were dressed in black, forming a half-circle around my bed. I am incredibly near-sighted and wear very thick glasses, so other than assuming the amorphous beings were human, I had no idea who they were. I started to drift back to sleep, but more chatter startled me into full attention, and I was suddenly terrified.

The combination of the narcotics, trauma, exhaustion, and near-sightedness made them appear so dark and shadowy. Was I overloaded with pain medicine and becoming delirious? I blinked several times to clear the sleep from my eyes and focused, glancing from side to side. No, I wasn't hallucinating. No less than five people were clustered around my bed, most of them dressed in black. This hospital assigned different classifications of employees to wear different colors, and the designation for RNs on this unit was black, which in my opinion, is a terrible color for *any* Nurse to wear. I tried to sit up when one of the figures reached out toward me.

Am I dead? I asked myself. *Who are these people, and why are they here?* "Who are you?" I asked, sincerely frightened. The memory of the accident came flooding back, and I wondered if I had died. However, my version of Heaven didn't come equipped with dark, shadowy figures, so I immediately stood firm on the conviction I was *not* dead but still among the living.

The figures came much closer until they were standing adjacent to the bed's rails. Despite my terrible vision, I recognized each of them as former students. They were all on duty on the Trauma or adjacent units. Never mind patient confidentiality, Dr. Foley was in the house, and apparently, word of my admission had spread quickly.

They hadn't tried to wake me but just stood there in disbelief and were trying to be as quiet as possible.

I first recognized Alex, a popular and attentive student who sat in the back row to the right of the podium. He had graduated two years before and had grown a beard, but I knew him immediately and called out his name: "Alex, back row podium right...sat with Brent, Sierra, and Brandon."

"That's it!" he said. "I can't believe you remember!" Nervous, relieved laughter spread across the room. Since most of them worked on the Trauma Unit, I suppose they wondered if I had suffered a closed head injury, knowing that some brain trauma doesn't become very evident until much later. "You look great, Alex. I hope the world of nursing is treating you well. My glasses please..." One of the other figures retrieved my glasses from a 'patient belongings bag' on the bedside table, and I was relieved they were so easily found. The lenses were streaked with blood, so Stacey, who I remembered as a kind, quiet student, took a moment to clean them while I lay cold, shivering, and in pain.

Students, a patient's 'appliances' or 'adaptive equipment' like dentures, hearing aids, and glasses are some of the most frequently lost items during hospital admissions. Please take great care when handling them.

Grateful to have mine, I again focused on these former students. I said their name, their classroom seating location, and the year they graduated. "OK folks, after that, you *know* I'm alert and oriented times four, right?" followed by some hearty laughs and a chorus of "is there anything else we can do for you? So sorry this happened. Everything will be ok."

Despite the pain, a feeling of comfort enveloped me. These students, who listened to my presentations on therapeutic communication, the stages of the Nurse-client relationship, locus of control, advocacy, interdisciplinary communication, and most importantly, the art and science of nursing, were standing in front of me as licensed professionals. Seeing them dressed in uniform made me feel like a proud parent. I fought off pain and drowsiness so I could seize this chance to talk to them. "Is nursing everything you thought it would be?" "Oh yeah," they replied, and one by one, they shared something about how their Nurse-Patient interactions brought to life concepts from various classes.

"Remember when we did those psych nursing simulations? They were great, and you were right. I have plenty of stories to tell myself. There *are* interesting patients everywhere you look," Allie offered. She looked very professional in her uniform and appeared so much more mature since she had graduated two years earlier. She seemed so pleased when I told her that, and after a few more pleasantries, the conversation quickly shifted to the expected "what happened...what brought you here?" questions.

Despite my circumstances, I thought clearly enough to filter the story a bit to salvage my pride. I couldn't admit my safety breach to them...not to my students, to whom I preached safety as a top priority so many times. Instead, I began to share my own experiences in Trauma

Bay 1. We all laughed, especially when I mentioned my interactions with the attending Physician they all apparently knew very well. "I hope you gave it to him good," Tyler said.

"I did my best in tribute to Nurses *everywhere*!" I said, followed by more laughter. Although tempted, I didn't mention the silver-haired male Nurse and his aberrant nursing practice. I did, however, extol the virtues of St. Vivian, for whom I had enormous respect. "Oh yeah, she's great," Alex said. "I've taken report from her a lot of times, and she definitely knows what she's doing."

I even allowed myself to tear up just a bit in front of them, and some of them teared up too. When I showed some genuine signs of pain and distress, they came to rapt attention and seemed alarmed, as though they were standing at a family member's bedside. I was so touched they all came to see me and didn't want the moment to tend. "You will all have to come back and have coffee with me at the University, or maybe we can all meet somewhere. I would like to hear all about your experiences in nursing. Have you thought about going back to school? There are so many great programs….." I must have fallen asleep, and when I woke up, they were gone. I wish I could have spoken with them so much longer to hear stories about their transition from student to practicing Nurse, but the narcotics won.

When I woke, I wondered if the delightful encounter had actually happened, but since many of them stopped in to check on me the next day, I was assured it had.

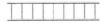

An undetermined amount of time had passed, and I realized two things: I was starving and had to urinate again. I pushed the call light, and to my amazement, Jonathan, one of my *current* students, was standing by my bedside in a white hospital uniform. He worked on this inpatient Trauma Unit as a Nursing Assistant and answered the call light. "I hope this isn't awkward for you, Dr. Foley. I volunteered to take care of you. I promise I will give you the highest quality care possible and assure you I am acting in a totally professional capacity and will observe all professional boundaries. Everything will remain confidential."

How impressive, Jonathan. Awkward, but impressive.

Despite some initial embarrassment on my part, I told him I needed only stand-by assistance. "Remember the Orem presentation from Nursing 101? You only have to be 'partially compensatory' for me." He smiled broadly and agreed. As one of my most outstanding students, I knew he would try his hardest to make the best of a potentially tricky situation. He went on to provide extraordinarily compassionate yet discrete care for the rest of the night. After another successful urination, I asked if I could sit in the chair, a request he happily accommodated. "Early ambulation has so many benefits, right Jonathan?" He agreed and helped me set up the dinner tray he thoughtfully reheated without being asked: pork roast, mashed potatoes, and vegetables.

Such a heavy meal was definitely out of the question, especially after blood, broken bones, X-rays, a CT scan, sedation, needles, sutures, but most of all, *that poor defunct silver-haired Nurse.*

Jonathan honored my request for a simple snack of ginger ale and some crackers. I still felt nauseous and recalled my father telling me that soda crackers were good for nausea, an old trick he learned in the Navy. Once they arrived, I realized my two-finger 'C' method might be suitable for urinating but was completely ineffective for eating. I couldn't open or pick up the can or the crackers, let alone manipulate silverware. My hands and fingers were imprisoned under loads of cotton padding and Ace wrap. I tried to call them into service several times, but their outgoing message said they were currently unavailable.

Oh no, someone would have to feed me.

As Jonathan put the first cracker into my mouth, I said, "you are continuing to be 'partially compensatory,' especially since my locus of control has been traumatically externalized.." On another occasion, I said, "you have done Jean Watson proud today as you demonstrate caring in its most practical form." He smiled and reminded me of his admiration for nursing theory and repeated the words I often spoke in class: "We have tasks to perform, but we must never become task-oriented." When he said good-bye at the end of his shift, I pointed out how effectively he engaged me throughout each stage of the Nurse-Patient relationship and joked about well he listened in class.

No, Jonathan, you are not task-oriented. Not one bit. Bravo. I wondered if he would discuss the care he provided with his classmates, but to my knowledge, he kept his promise and never did. Double bravo, Jonathan.

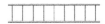

Despite these uplifting experiences with students, the first night still presented many challenges. The Orthopedic Residents placed an order to elevate my arms vertically inside two large rectangles of pink foam. No one ever told me the technical name of these torture devices, but I despised them. I intellectually understood their purpose—to protect my arms and to minimize the chance of dependent edema (swelling that can occur when a limb is in a downward position). Nevertheless, they were quite top-heavy, and each time I drifted off to sleep, one of my arms would tip over, causing excruciating pain. After calling out a few times, I finally didn't ask but *told* a Nursing Assistant I hadn't met before to free my arms and elevate them on two pillows. The Orthopedic Residents weren't too pleased when they made rounds, but I told them it was my decision and took full responsibility. A quick shrug, and they were on their way.

After that, I slept soundly for several more hours.

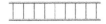

I woke up to see Ellen standing over me, just in time to help me with a late breakfast. It seemed so odd to have a sibling feed me. She is six years older than me and babysat me quite a bit when we were small children, but now, this act of caring seemed awkward in adulthood. I was nevertheless very grateful. We never spoke while she fed me and didn't resume our usual brother-sister banter until we were *both* sitting down and preparing to indulge in a cup of coffee, our go-to beverage of choice. She brought a large coffee from the snack bar downstairs and offered to split it with me. How wonderful! No tepid hospital coffee for me, but I had to consume my treat through a straw.

We both carefully avoided discussing the previous day's events because, honestly, I don't think we were prepared to discuss them just yet. We chose instead to address the elephant-in-the-living-room topic: when we were going to tell our parents. "It's Friday, and mom will be expecting to come to my house tomorrow. I will tell her something came up, and she can come over on Sunday instead."

It has been a tradition in my family that my mom came to my house at 9 am on Saturdays. After coffee and conversation, we usually do a bit of shopping and have lunch, returning to my house for more coffee and dessert after that. I knew how much she looked forward to the weekly visits. "Mom is going to be very upset. Maybe we should tell her tonight."

Although I knew she was right, nonetheless, I stood my ground. "I suspect I will be discharged on Sunday morning, and she can come over to my house then. We can visit on Sunday instead of Saturday. I don't know what I'm going to do once I get home. I am going to need help around the house. Everyone will just have to come and see me for a while because I can't travel….."

BILL!!!!!!

My closest human and brother-from-another-mother was vacationing in Las Vegas and didn't know what had happened. I had known him for many years, and we had shared the best and worst of our lives. He is one of those people who gives to others unselfishly, no matter what the cost. An extremely dynamic and popular guy, he had recently been diagnosed with a chronic health condition that forced him to take early retirement and make some drastic changes to his active lifestyle. His vacation had been in the works for many months, and I was tempted not to call him until he returned home, but then remembered he was returning home tomorrow. "Ellen, you better call Bill. He will be mad if he isn't told. I hate to ruin the last day of his vacation, though."

My sister dialed his number and put the phone to my ear, intently avoiding my gaze. I tried to turn my head away, insisting she make the call, but Bill, recognizing my number, answered on the second ring. I had no choice to tell him. "Are you sitting down?" I began and tried to laugh in a genuine, carefree manner. "What's wrong?" Bill asked me, knowing I would likely not disturb him on vacation if it wasn't good news.

I told him of my condition in the most economical manner possible. He listened intently and said, "I'll be there Sunday." I protested but knew it would do no good. As I've often said, you have family, and you have *family,* and as a result of his selfless, caring nature, he falls within the latter category. I told him I thought I might come home on Sunday but wasn't sure, so we agreed to talk on Saturday after his flight landed and go from there. In addition to my sister's support, knowing someone cared enough to travel two and half hours to help me was incredibly meaningful and gave me some needed strength. The visit would be no fun whatsoever, but I knew he would be okay with that.

Yes, Bill was coming, and that meant more help was on the way.

PART IV

ONE DAY IN SAFETY

CHAPTER 11

A BEAUTIFUL MOSAIC

Today, the world can appear fragmented and its people disconnected. Mosaics allow me to **fuse the pieces together to create something cohesive and beautiful, what I wish the world could be.**
Laura Harris

FORMER—AND CURRENT—STUDENTS FILTERED in and out of my room over the next two days, sometimes as my assigned Registered Nurse, other times as my Nursing Assistant, and sometimes just to say hello. Despite two broken arms, with so much support, I quickly learned to be as independent as possible and was relieved I *could* feed and toilet myself...

well, almost. It was truly amazing—and very enlightening—how such small victories added to my sense of empowerment as I enthusiastically partnered with anyone willing to help move my locus of control just a tiny bit closer.

I received care from many people other than former students, however. Nurses who staffed this hospital were graduates of schools scattered across the metropolitan area and beyond, hailing from diploma, associate's, and bachelor's degree programs. They created a delightful mosaic of our area's best and finest caregivers and beautifully captured many dimensions of diversity, the hopeful spirit of my dissertation. In particular, three nurses captured my attention, creating a trifecta of the factors that embodied the subjects of that research: Nurses who are male, of color, or with limited English proficiency (LEP). Receiving top-quality nursing care from them was highly validating.

In hindsight, I realized providing care to me, an experienced Nurse and nursing instructor, may not have been easy. At various points during my hospital stay, I reflected on my own needs, especially concerning my own psychosocial assessment, which entailed my current developmental stage and psycho-social status. Deep in thought, I asked myself how *a Nurse colleague would demonstrate culturally competent care to me, a 50-year-old devout Christian Caucasian male who just happened to* be a doctorally-prepared Nurse Educator. What exactly *was* my cultural framework, and how might it impact relationships with my caregivers and, ultimately, my care? I continually preached to my nursing students to "look below the dotted line" of their assessment sheet's physical findings to understand how spiritual, social, cultural, and psychological factors may impact a patient's response to treatment. With nothing better to do, I chose to do a self-assessment using Erikson'sStages of Psychosocial Development as a framework for analysis. The task proved surprisingly difficult, but after much deliberation, I came up with the following:

Age:	50 years old
Developmental Stage:	Generativity vs. Stagnation
Ethnicity:	Anglo-Saxon (English and Irish)
Religion:	Christian (devout and practicing)
Education:	PhD (Education-Nursing Education; with other advanced degrees in nursing and administration)
Profession:	University professor and Nurse
Economic Status:	Comfortable
Health:	Adequate health-seeking behaviors with excellent insurance
Social:	Extensive, supportive social network

After much thought, I concluded I was very blessed with many resources that would aid my recovery. I was also very engaged in my care and doing my best to be a compliant patient. On the other hand, based on my educational background, I decided I might also be a problematic patient…to say the least. I had already demonstrated that in the parking lot by resolving to 'go undercover,' which proved to be a successful coping strategy until my 'may I have your attention please?' outburst directed at the Trauma Bay's Physician.

Oops. I can only imagine what kind of nursing report Vivian provided to 5B Nurse Tina. "He's a handful. You should have heard what he said to Dr.…." Knowing how Nurses talk, maybe *that's* why so many of my former students heard I was in the hospital. I read somewhere that Physicians make the worst patients. Although I agree with that notion to a point, I also think many Nurses and other interdisciplinary team members also make terrible patients. Perhaps I (and the collective 'we') just can't help ourselves.

With that thought in mind, I decided to delve deeply into my thoughts on resolving Erikson's Stage of Psychosocial Development called Generativity vs. Stagnation/Self-Absorption. I recalled this involved the period between the early 40s and mid-60s where adults attempt to nurture and create things that will outlast them. Although I've never had children, I realized I have helped many students achieve academic success and transition into practice.

Did that count? I hoped so.

Progress at resolving Generativity vs. Stagnation/ Self-Absorption can be assessed in one question: How have I contributed to the world? I think that question was resolved a little bit at a time as each student or group of students stopped by to see me at the bedside and, as I was soon to experience, visited me at home.

I must admit I had actively avoided a personal developmental or psycho-social stage assessment for a long time. In class, I encouraged students to assess their own stage and steps toward resolution but realized I might have been reluctant to do so.

Had I contributed to the world? Thanks to the concern and countless acts of caring demonstrated by my students, I came to the conclusion I had. The attribute 'care' is assigned to the stage of Generativity vs. Stagnation. As a person who is a firm believer of Faith in action, I decided was I had been successful in demonstrating caring toward many patients and hundreds of students who will carry on a collective legacy of caring far into the future.

Self-assessment completed.

Generativity vs. Stagnation/Self-Absorption on its way to successful resolution.

I must admit if there was one positive aspect of being hospitalized, it was those realizations. Laying there, I chose to continue my legacy even by encouraging the staff caring for me, some of whom were already in school while others were still contemplating the idea.

Yes, I confess I meddled in my care, acted in a very stealthy manner to expedite my discharge, and watched anything and everything around me through the eyes of a trained compliance surveyor. Nonetheless, I think the most satisfying part of my hospital stay (if there was one) was being cared for by a group of incredibly talented and delightfully diverse Nurses.

Without realizing it (and no…it wasn't just due to the haze of pain and narcotics), I guess I resolved to cope by asking my caregivers about their own educational experiences and backgrounds and encouraging them to continue their education. After all, I had spent several years gearing up for doctoral work and then four full years enmeshed in the dissertation process itself. Why not put it to good use?

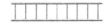

Sophia

Like so many other recent immigrants from Eastern Europe, Sophia and her immediate family pounced on easing travel restrictions and visited the United States just after the collapse of the former Soviet Union. They were captivated by what they saw and choose to emigrate, settling in our metropolitan area in 2009. A highly skilled Surgeon in her own country, Sophia decided not to pursue a career in medicine in the United States. Sadly, I'd heard this story several times before from many other immigrants who were Physicians in their homeland. The task of relearning the entirety of the medical curriculum well enough to pass the US Medical Board Examination was too overwhelming, especially given the concurrent linguistic challenge of mastering English.

I could undoubtedly commiserate because much of the material I learned in nursing school proved useful only to pass the NCLEX-RN and was then promptly forgotten. Once Nurses enter practice, much foundational knowledge, especially in courses like Obstetrics and Pediatrics, is simply not needed for everyday practice unless, of course, a Nurse self-selects into one of those specialties. I couldn't imagine moving to another country where English is not spoken, let alone relearning all the required nursing curriculum well enough to pass the NCLEX-RN in a foreign language. I immediately felt much empathy for her.

Sophia made a brave, resolute choice to leave medicine behind and become a Nursing Assistant in the United States. She told me it meant infinitely more to raise her children in this country than keep her status as a Physician within a government system she could no longer support. When she introduced herself, she appeared a bit nervous, so it was apparent at least one of the other Nurses had told her I was a nursing professor. I broke the ice by asking her what led her into nursing. She told me it was incredibly humbling to transition from Physician to Nursing Assistant, but her inability to speak English was the real hindrance.

Nevertheless, she had to start somewhere. She and her husband worked very hard at their respective jobs during the day. They then supported each other in learning English in the evening, vowing to take coursework in America as soon as they achieved command of the English language.

After one year of intense study, Sophia took the Test of English as Foreign Language (TOEFL) exam and scored well enough to be placed on the waiting list for an Associates Degree in Nursing Program at a local community college. She went to school during the day and worked in the evening. Her husband, an engineer by trade, also returned to school, but she never disclosed his new career. She did, however, convey with pride that they had worked very hard to establish themselves in America.

Sophia made eye contact with me very few times during our many interactions, and I wondered if her avoidance of eye contact was based on cultural factors. Later that day, one of my former students was on duty and spoke very highly of Sophia. Smiling, he validated that I made her nervous since word had spread I was a teacher, and she didn't want to disappoint me.

Sophia cared for me that day and the next. I encouraged her as much as I could to return to school to pursue graduate studies in nursing. I even offered to put her in touch with my good friend, now a Nurse Practitioner, who also had a previous career as a non-English speaking professional in her home country. Sophia was hard working, had excellent follow-through, and exuded professionalism through her work and demeanor. I sincerely hoped she would consider going back to school.

Unlike Sophia, many of my former students with LEP were not successful in completing their pre-licensure nursing programs. They often failed in the pivotal first or second semesters, that stressful time when the onslaught of nursing-medical terminology collided with the ongoing challenges of mastering English. As one of my dissertation's recommendations, I suggested helping such 'at risk' students through early intervention at the first sign of difficulty during that first semester and by allowing them to identify their strengths and weaknesses *before* admission to the nursing program.

I recalled many inspirational scenes walking through the nursing building and seeing students with limited English proficiency (LEP) nursing from various countries across the globe huddled together and studying with quiet intensity. Although their countries of origin were different, they stood unified in achieving program completion despite the linguistic challenge. They formed unlikely yet enduring friendships across age, ethnic, geographic, political, and religious lines.

Sophia listened very intently while I encouraged her to go back to school. It was the only time she looked me directly in the eye, and I hoped the encouragement validated her skills and abilities. I told her to please move forward and that I just "knew" she could do it. Sophia smiled, nodded, and moved on with her work.

As a tiny yet tangible demonstration of my efforts to be culturally competent, I have taken pride in learning a few words in many different languages. Luckily, I knew a few in Russian and peppered them throughout the conversation. In those moments, Sophia smiled and laughed.

Cultural competence is a foundational concept of transcultural nursing. The prefix 'trans' means across, so the term means making active attempts to reach across actual or perceived cultural barriers as an integral part of the nursing process. In doing so, Nurses can provide care to patients within their own cultural frame of reference. It felt very fulfilling to receive care from a Nurse who hailed from another culture, and the experience strengthened my resolve to support LEP students in the future.

I never anticipated I would reflect on Transcultural Nursing from the patient's perspective. Still, I sensed that working together, Sophia and I made Madeleine Leininger and her Culture Care Theory proud. Sophia, I hope you return to school very soon. Your community—and the community at large—needs many more talented Nurses like you.

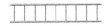

Randy

Anyone who resides in my closest inner circle of friends and family has heard schadenfreude from my own experiences during nursing school. Strict, overly disciplined nursing instructors who were mistreated in nursing school were more than pleased to pass along the favor to us unsuspecting students. Such 'tragic' stories are a theme offered by many nursing students, but for me, a *male* nursing student, they took on a special meaning.

Yes, I can attest that Nurses eat their young.

So many colleagues related their stories of becoming nauseous before clinicals, having panic attacks before classroom exams, or nearly passing out during skills test-outs in the nursing resource lab. Such challenges are complex for Caucasian females, who comprise the majority of nursing students. Yet, I often ask students and colleagues alike to consider how difficult it was for those of us—myself included—who fell outside the majority's safety net.

From the start of my nursing school experience, I felt marginalized and alone. I was often the only male in some of my nursing classes and the *only* male in smaller clinical groups. I knew something was wrong but hadn't yet gained the knowledge or perspective to know what to call it. Later as I devoured article after article in my master's program, I realized the enormous influence an instructor's implicit—or explicit—bias could have on a nursing student's emerging professional identity.

According to many sources, it would seem many men hunker down and then fall into a very predictable pattern of self-selecting into nursing's crisis-oriented or 'technical' disciplines like Emergency Medicine, Critical Care, Life Flight, or the Operating Room. Sadly, this means they also shy *away from* nursing's 'softer disciplines' like Obstetrics or Pediatrics. Even quite recently, I've had young male nursing students tell me practicing Nurses, both female and male, have discouraged them from pursuing a career within specific disciplines in nursing. "You won't find a job," one established Nurse said and then elaborated, "Be practical. That's not a career for men. They will make your life miserable." The ubiquitous 'they,' still influencing men to pursue a career path in nursing that is gender-based, socially appropriate, and perhaps in their eyes, even biologically pre-determined.

One of my first orders of business as a nursing instructor was to encourage *all* students to pursue the path—any path—in nursing that inspired them. I came to peace long ago that a Florence Nightingale-esque noble, altruistic calling into the profession is simply no longer a motivating factor for many of them. Instead, many male and female students enter the profession as a pathway to social and economic mobility, especially given the departure of our geographic area's manufacturing base and unfortunate designation as a 'rust belt' state. Nevertheless, after entry into practice, I sincerely hoped they would fall in love with the profession just as I had many years earlier.

Such was the apparent case with Randy, a very congenial young man who came into my room, looked me squarely in the eye, and declared he would be my Nurse for the day shift. I knew that male nursing students, like other minorities, often fall prey to a mighty foe—attrition (or program failure) rates that are usually at least twice as high as their female counterparts. Since men comprise only about nine percent of the nursing workforce, having one as my Nurse felt very validating.

Randy efficiently reviewed my vital signs and labs and then discussed my plan of care. He assessed my comfort and breezed through my list of medications. He even asked if I had eaten my breakfast. None of these acts were particularly impressive or noble, but I just took note this young Nurse seemed to be covering all the basics in a very efficient manner.

Of course, I asked Randy where he went to school and about his future aspirations. He said he had found his niche in critical care nursing and was returning to school to become a Nurse Practitioner. "Is that really what you want?" I couldn't help but ask him. "Yeah, it really is," he quickly replied. "Heroes have always inspired me. My dad was a medic in the army, and this is as close as I can come to following in his footsteps." I briefly asked him about nursing school, and he didn't convey anything but positive experiences.

Good. I hope things are changing.

Randy's care was thoughtfully deliberate. He used clean technique when administering my medications and made sure I was comfortably positioned before he left the room. As it turned out, Randy also knew I was a professor of nursing, and I wondered if that impacted how he cared for me.

I decided I didn't think so. A Nurse can't make up the style of ease, and efficiency Randy displayed. He seemed very confident in his nursing practice, and I don't believe someone could craft such a satisfying impression on the spot. He was comfortable in his nursing skin, which was evident by his easy, confident communication and fluent practice.

Randy gave me a lot of inspiration that day. I hoped progress was being made in terms of males gaining a foothold within the profession of nursing. Randy didn't arrive at this place alone. Kudos to those who helped him arrive at such a rich and comfortable place within the profession.

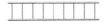

Within the metropolitan area surrounding the hospital lies a highly intricate network of neighborhoods and suburbs with varying levels of diversity. However, in certain sections of my mental map, only a distance of one mile would mean crossing a boundary separating highly segregated areas with very different socio-economic statuses and vastly different educational experiences. These factors were of great interest to me as an educator and heavily influenced my teaching and research.

As a result, the last group I focused on in my dissertation was students of color. Our surrounding urban area is nearly sixty percent minority, yet the student composition in my classes is usually less than 10%. Thanks to those infamous attrition rates, actual graduation rates for students of color often fell below 5%.

Growing up in the 1970s, I witnessed firsthand the growing social consciousness regarding the shameful practices of segregation in our local school systems, and I vowed to do what I could to create a learning experience that was as inclusive and culturally sensitive as possible. Based on differences in socioeconomic status and educational backgrounds, I recognized students came to nursing school with widely varying amounts of social capital, or the cultural knowledge and social connections to succeed. These were the same thoughts I had about being a male in nursing, as my female Nurse colleagues shared common experiences that I did not.

Despite my status as a Caucasian male, as a student nurse, I found myself having more in common with the few students of color and the students with LEP than the Caucasian females, who constituted over 90 percent of my graduating class.

I cannot portray myself as a noble humanitarian. I simply want to promote the success of each of my students so the nursing workforce may look just a bit more like our surrounding community. In my opinion, a more diverse workforce adds to nursing's collective cultural competence, and that will surely enhance our area's standard of care. I worked with other faculty and students to re-invigorate a fledgling chapter of a minority student Nurse group. I enjoyed our meetings where, despite our outward differences, we could all celebrate our experience, strength, and hope in the profession of nursing.

In a similar manner to my male and LEP students, I monitored the progress of my students of color very closely. I watched many of them display a reluctance to ask for help until academic failure was imminent; I quickly decided I could not stand passively by and watch that happen. From the podium's unique perspective, I could clearly see students who were isolated, quiet, and floundering. I asked a number of them if I could introduce them to another supportive student, only later to receive an email later telling me it helped. Sometimes the pairing involved a cultural match, while other times not, but that really didn't matter. The introductions were intended only to introduce two people in hopes they may provide each other with some badly needed support.

Flash forward to the school's annual nursing pinning ceremony, where students proudly walked across the stage to receive their nursing pin and rounds of applause from their colleagues, family, and loved ones. Students were allowed to pick a faculty member of their choice to 'pin' them, typically someone who inspired them or encouraged them to succeed. Based on their requests, I was asked to be a 'head pinner' for two years in a row. It was enormously challenging to hold back tears as the students approached me to receive their pin while their families cheered—and cried—in the audience.

I truly believed we were making progress.

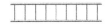

Kara

My Nursing Assistant for this shift was Kara, a lovely young African American woman with an engaging smile and pleasant demeanor. Of course, I asked her where she was attending nursing school. "How did you know I was in school?" she asked. I told her I just knew—she had 'the look,' and we both laughed. She said she was enrolled in the local community college's Associate Degree in Nursing Program and was hoping to graduate next year.

Hoping? Tell me more, Kara.

She shared that she was previously enrolled in another local school's Bachelor of Science in Nursing program. She was unsuccessful in a course during her junior year, one of the classes with a notorious reputation for student failures. Kara told me she tried very hard to earn a high enough grade on the final exam to earn a passing grade but failed by two points.

Yuk.

Thinking it might be easier, or at the very least, less costly, Kara chose to enroll in the local community college's Associate Degree in Nursing Program. Attracted by their promises of immediate admission but scared away by the exorbitant cost, she had briefly considered a few of the local proprietary schools' nursing programs. "I already have a lot of student loans from my other school. I couldn't imagine adding another 40, possibly 50 thousand dollars to my debt, so I picked the Associate Degree Program, where the tuition is much less expensive. I know I'll need to go on and get my BSN at some point, but at least I can be earning a living while I do it."

When I asked her how she was doing in her new program, Kara said she was "…getting by but nervous about an upcoming exam. I thought it might be easier, but it really isn't. It's the same material that made me fail at my other school." Kara also shared she wanted to graduate to get a better job and give her two-year-old daughter the best possible life. "I want to show her mommy *can do it.*"

"Yes, Kara, you can do it.!" I told her. I believed that because I had seen others do it many times before. Despite impossible work schedules, differences in social capital, LEP, and instructor bias, they created a support system, attacked their stressors, and persevered. Kara said she wanted to eventually work as a Nurse Practitioner, more than likely in family practice. "I took this Nursing Assistant job because I thought it would help prepare me to work wherever I land."

That sounds like a great plan, Kara, and I believe you will land squarely on your feet.

I really respected Kara. She was one of those caregivers who made negotiating any perceived or actual cultural divide easy; she simply embodied how to 'do' cultural competence. I could tell she was very secure with her own identity, and that made addressing the needs of others within their own space so much easier.

Kara represented another large group of students for whom I also had much admiration: working-class, single parent, and 'non-traditional' students. In her early 30's, Kara demonstrated a level of maturity and responsibility beyond her years, and I admired that.

She provided me with excellent care and instinctively knew when to offer help, then telescope back to let me try on my own. As a cheerleader and motivator, she also provided 'standby' assistance while I walked to the restroom, then sensed my modesty and closed the door to give privacy and gave words of encouragement when I was able to "go on my own." Although I can't say for sure, I doubt this motivated, personable nursing student contributed to *her* new school of nursing's attrition rates. I have to believe she has graduated and is now in practice, contemplating a return to school to pursue graduate studies. In my optimistic world, that's certainly the way it should be.

I wish you the best, Kara.

The Grand Finale: Thomas

As I dozed that evening, I opened my eyes to see another figure dressed in black standing next to my bed. I was startled and called out, "who are you?" As soon as I spoke the words, I focused and recognized precisely who the figure was: a wonderfully articulate and compassionate former student—now recent graduate— named Thomas. Thomas was a male student of color and a second-generation immigrant for whom English was a second language.

All three in one fantastic package!

"I'm so sorry, Professor Foley! I didn't mean to scare you. Are you doing ok? Is there anything I can get for you?" He smiled warmly as he spoke, feet planted firmly on the ground, making eye contact with me. "Thanks Thomas," I replied. "I see your attempts to initiate an effective Nurse-Patient relationship. Did you ever think it would be with me?"

"No," he said, "never. But really though, can I get you anything?"

"Not right at the moment. How are things going for you? Did you take the NCLEX-RN yet?" Thomas was one of my better students, and I assumed he had already taken the exam and likely passed, but past lessons taught me never to assume. After students graduate in May, the school must send a Program Completion Letter to the Board of Nursing advising them a student has successfully fulfilled all requirements prescribed by the school's curriculum. Once received, the State Board usually takes a few weeks to review the letters and issue the student a 'notification of permission to test,' after which they may schedule their appointment with an approved testing site and take their exam.

This timeline means the vast majority of nursing graduates take the NCLEX-RN and achieve licensure by the end of August, and since this was now September, I assumed he had already passed. Students can pay extra to have their results expedited and not endure the interminable wait I experienced when I graduated nearly twenty years earlier. Adding to the stress, job offers from area hospitals are often conditional and subject to successfully passing the NCLEX-RN.

As if he read my mind, Thomas interrupted my thoughts. "I passed Boards at the end of August, and I'm now orienting to this floor. I asked your Nurse if I could come in and check on you."

"Of course you passed, Thomas. I had no doubt you would. You were always a star." I paused as he smiled and seemed a bit embarrassed. "Do you remember when you met with me during your first semester in school? You asked me for tips on how to succeed in nursing school. It looks like you're doing so well you should be giving other students tips on how to succeed. I hope we can have you come back and speak to future classes."

Thomas' wife worked in an ancillary health profession, and they both decided quite pragmatically they would live on her salary while Thomas attended nursing school. Though only in his mid-20's, he had a sense of maturity and professionalism that far exceeded his years.

As I had witnessed many times, the story was often not nearly as bright for other male nursing students.

Although men are being admitted to nursing programs in higher numbers, the attrition rates for male students are also often much higher than those for females. In turn, if a group of men was admitted to a cohort, by graduation, some of them voluntarily exited and selected another major or were not academically successful, forcing them to withdraw from the nursing program.

Thomas was hardly at risk to add to the attrition rates in his class. He was thoughtfully inquisitive and was never afraid to display caring behaviors within his self-concept of masculinity. I remembered how he remained at rapt attention during class, even when some of the content was, well, a bit dry. Thomas embodied the notion 'people who act enthusiastic will be enthusiastic!' Throughout the program, I never heard him complain— not even once. He was resilient and viewed challenges as opportunities, including caring for his former instructor on this evening shift.

"Are you my Nurse, Thomas?"

"No, but that's ok. I volunteered to come in and help you. I'm orienting, so I have some time on my hands. What can I do for you?" Thomas asked quietly. "Can you help me up so I can go to the restroom? I don't need any help other than getting up. I can do the rest myself," I quickly offered.

"It's ok if you do need help," Thomas soothed, "Professors sometimes need help too."

I watched as Thomas made sure the bed was locked, adjusted the head of my bed to a High Fowler's position, and carefully lowered the side rails. "Ok Professor Foley, let's take it slow," as he delicately pulled down the blanket and sheets. "Let's sit on the side of the bed for a minute so you can get used to the change. You're taking pain medications and have been through a trauma, so you don't need to move too quickly. No falls tonight."

"OK, Thomas," I told him, smiling weakly.

I got up slowly with stand-by assistance and shuffled carefully to the bathroom. I quickly used my "C" method to pull back my hospital gown, luckily having just enough strength so I could also pull back my briefs and urinate. I even managed to flush the toilet myself by pushing the button with my foot.

Thomas smiled as I celebrated my bathroom victory. "I performed an activity of daily living with just stand-by assistance, Thomas. Woo hoo." We both laughed as I got back in bed. After a while, I opened my eyes to find him gone. I had no idea what time it was, but I assumed it was the middle of the night, and I sensed I had slept for maybe two hours. I thought about Thomas and many other students, hoping I had encouraged them to forge a positive nursing identity free from gender—or any— bias. "Be whichever kind of Nurse you want," I told them, "but be sure to find ways to be compassionate. No matter who you are, provide top quality, compassionate, patient-centered care anywhere you go in the continuum of care."

Thomas did just that, and in the darkness of that room with pain as my constant companion, I couldn't help but compare Thomas' interpersonal style, use of therapeutic communication, and nursing skills with some of the other Nurses I encountered during my career.

Thanks to great students like Thomas, I sensed the future for men in nursing was bright. "Thank you, Thomas," I thought as I lapsed into sleep, deeply regretting the narcotics had once again robbed me of spending more time with him.

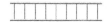

The Residents

A Nurse's relationship with a Resident is one that slowly evolves over time. Each July, the atmosphere within the hospital is quite chaotic, as the first-year Residents, initially buoyantly optimistic and full of confidence, quickly realize they have much to learn. For them, eustress indeed does become distress too. As an unspoken cultural norm, Nurses give the new batch of Residents some time to prove themselves. Although there is a sense of tacit acknowledgment of the roles in the Nurse-Resident relationship, from the outset, a Nurse can easily withdraw respect based on a Resident's perceived lack of confidence, incompetence, or worse yet, incivility. Whether we realize it or not, Nurses play a vital role in a Resident's education. For example, Nurses can question a new Resident's written orders, quickly forcing them out of their perceived state of unconscious competence (better known as 'I think I know a great deal, but I don't') and to the next stop on the competence continuum: conscious incompetence (better known as the 'the veil has been ripped off and I know nothing').

There are situations when time constraints—and patient acuity—don't support discrete communication and I've seen many Nurses publically remind a new Resident of the need to rethink a decision or check a medication order. Based on the new Resident's response, the Nurse will adjust the relationship accordingly: a Resident who takes feedback in stride is considered to be reasonable and approachable, while Residents who become angry, defensive, or even hostile will find their names entered onto an unwritten, unofficial naughty list that quickly circulates by word of mouth. Depending on the Resident's offense, I have even witnessed Nurses conspire to keep them up all night when they are on call. They accomplish this by resolving to "...bother them for every little thing, including acetaminophen." If and when the Resident repents, the Nurses will reassess and move them to the 'reasonable and approachable list' as soon as they start cooperating.

All in a days' work.

I looked forward to watching the Residents' inter-actions with the nursing staff to determine if they were on the 'good' list. I also suspected the Residents who cared for me in Trauma Bay 1 were very new, as they seemed aloof and uncommunicative, perhaps as a defense mechanism to shield their lack of experience or skill.

For example, the Orthopedic Residents did not support my hand properly (which to me seemed like common sense), resulting in a loud chastisement from the attending Physician and the Plastic Surgery. The Residents thus seemed incapable of independent thought, taking every cue from their senior Resident.

Yikes. Maybe they're all new!

At any rate, a different group of Orthopedic Residents stopped by my room around 2 am and woke me from a sound sleep to check on my progress. My progress? Interesting choice of words, especially since only a little more than a day had elapsed since my accident. Since I could not feed myself, I grilled them about why my left arm had been wrapped so aggressively. When would the Attending be stopping by to do his assessment and possibly grant my fingers a bit of clemency? "We're sorry about that, one of them told me, but we wanted to be aggressive with wrapping them to prevent any more injury."

"When will the attending be stopping by?"

"We'll get to that in a minute. How is your pain level?"

I was trying to take as few pain medications as possible, first because my pain level was manageable, and second, because I thought I had become overly sedated the night before. In fact, at one point, I saw tiny points of light dancing in my peripheral field of vision and was sure I was becoming delirious. I accordingly declined the last round of pain medications that were offered to me just two hours prior.

"Right now, my pain's OK," I told them. Can I go home today?"

"No, not today. If all goes well, you can go home tomorrow or the day after so you can rest up before your surgery on Tuesday."

"SURGERY? WHAT SURGERY?" I called out, absolutely incredulous.

One of the group, a small, petite young female Resident, moved forward half a step and said, "You need surgery on your right arm. We did our best to stabilize it in the Emergency Department, but you need surgery to insert a metal plate with such a bad break. We're Orthopedics, but the Plastic Surgery Hand service will do your surgery because they were on call the day of your accident. The Plastics Hand Team will be making rounds later, and they can give you more specifics."

"So you're not following my case?" *Then why did you bother me by so late? I was sleeping so well…*

"Sort of. We still round on all orthopedic cases since this is a teaching hospital."

"Oh. Well, are you *sure* I'm going to have surgery next week? Maybe the Plastics Hand Team's attending will think I won't need surgery. When will they be stopping by…"

The Resident smiled and said she doubted that would be the case. I asked them while they were there if they would *please* try to re-wrap my arms so I could have a bit more use of my fingers? Again, they said they could not. Ask 'Plastics Hand' was their reply. They would be around later to see me. With that, they turned around and scurried quietly out of the room, their paper shoe protectors making a soft, swishing sound against the tile floor. Why hadn't the team Trauma Bay 1 or one of my Nurses told me about the surgery? I couldn't imagine going home and returning to this place for another painful procedure. Logic quickly prevailed, and I surmised such a 'gross deformity' would need more aggressive intervention than just a cast. On a more optimistic note, I guessed the surgery would be outpatient, so I could at least go home immediately following.

Later, around 3 am, I was once again in a sound sleep when a Plastics Hand Resident arrived to inform me the severity of the break in my right forearm required surgical intervention. As I peered at her sleepily, she said she also had good news: the break in my *left* wrist didn't need surgery but would require a hard cast for 7-10 weeks.

That's good news? Well, I guess it is...

She further related there was still some debate among the team if the left Triquetral (wrist) fracture would require surgery in the future. Still, she was cautiously optimistic it would heal with the benefit of casting alone. Could Plastics Hand (by this time, I stopped thinking of the Residents as people and referred to them by their service) please partially re-wrap my fingers so I could have a bit more mobility? No, they could not do that either, at least not now. My surgery was on Tuesday. All wraps and dressings would be removed in the presence of the attending Surgeon just before the procedure, who would review the X-rays and decide how aggressive any permanent casting, splinting, and wrapping would be. In the meantime, I was to be patient and get some rest. She was direct but polite, and although tempted to argue, I realized my frustration shouldn't be taken out on him.

OK, I guess you don't have much choice, and Tuesday is right around the corner. I just hoped they don't call to cancel or reschedule this surgery. I want it over as soon as possible...

After she left, my mind forcibly shut down from complete exhaustion *(I mean, geez, can't Residents make their rounds before bedtime?),* and I fell into a deep sleep. I woke up at 9 am to see Sophia standing over me with her gentle smile. "Hello, sleepyhead," she said, her accent sounding so poetic. "I think I have some good news. Your team is thinking of discharging you later today, but probably not until the late afternoon or early evening, depending on how things go."

"Today? But I thought...." trailing off to a peaceful, silent smile.

Woo hoo. I'm going home! Try not to act too excited, but let's do this! I knew exactly what I had to do to get out of here: show I can stand, walk, eat, make attempts to care for myself, and remind them I have a robust support system in place.

"Sophia, I'm going to get up and use the restroom. I feel like walking, and I'm hungry. Will breakfast be here soon? I'd like to eat before my family and friends arrive."

Slow down, Nurse Foley...

PART V

THREE DAYS IN SAFETY

CHAPTER 12

HOME, JAMES

Getting out of the hospital is a lot like resigning from a book club. You're not out of it until the computer says you're out of it.
Erma Bombeck

HERE, LET ME help you. Please be careful. I'll have someone heat up your breakfast," Sophia interjected, but there was no stopping me. I carefully planted my feet on the floor, being very mindful to wait a few moments to avoid a sudden postural change and possible syncopal (fainting) episode. I noted Sophia was carefully monitoring my gait and ability to walk independently, one of the critical activities of daily living.

She made every effort to perform an accurate physical and mental status assessment, and I cooperated to the max. "I just feel like walking, Sophia. I think it will be good for me, don't you?"

She seemed momentarily surprised as I slowly headed for the door. "Be careful, David," her accent sounding even more melodic than before. "Oh, I plan on it, Sophia," I called back, and *just watch me go home today...I'm getting out of here!* The Trauma Unit was contained within a round tower, with each floor's hallway forming a perfect circle with the Nurses' station in the center. Having sat in on many building design sessions in my career, I could almost hear the architects and builders going over the rationale for the design: "Having the Nurses' station in the center will allow the Nurses to keep a continuous watch on the entire floor...." Imagination aside, I realized the circle provided me the perfect stage to put on my show. I would walk around several times with a deliberate, careful gait so all could see the progress I had made in such short order.

Only then would I retreat to my room to eat and toilet myself and, as a grand finale, actually attempt to comb my hair using my "C hook" method.
- Ambulation....check
- Transfer in and out of bed....check
- Eating and drinking...check
- Grooming....semi-check
- Toileting....semi-check

- Dressing….no
- Motivation….check, check
- Strong support system…check, check, check!!!

Would it be enough to impress my interdisciplinary team well enough to secure my release? I hoped so.

Shortly after that, the Trauma Team made rounds, and I eyed them nervously while they interviewed me. I patiently answered their questions and calmly told them I had a caring, intact family unit and lived in a one-story ranch-style home with no steps. I felt confident I would be cared for in an environment that was safe and secure.

While they were speaking, a group of smiling friends crowded into the room, carrying flowers and gifts. *Right on cue…thank you!* Without saying another word, I smiled at the Team, and the spokesperson said, "well, let's see if we can get you out of here today. It may take a while, but I think you can go home. Just be patient."

The visit with my friends was cheerful and optimistic. Despite the gnawing, aching pain that was still my constant unwelcomed companion, I made a firm decision that I would take only Acetaminophen and avoid narcotics. Instead, I used ice packs, deep breathing and relaxation, and guided imagery as often as possible, which seemed to help quite a bit. Although I had instructed many patients to use those alternative pain management strategies, I now understood their limitations and, in the future, would speak about them from a far more personal and informed perspective.

Early that evening, none other than Sophia presented to my room with my discharge paperwork. She smiled shyly as she went over the instructions saying, "I'm sure you can read all of this on your own but as a formality..."

"Oh no, Sophia, I appreciate you going over the instructions with me. Please go on."

When she was finished, I called my sister, who arrived to take me home within an hour. Despite my protests, Sophia insisted on wheeling me to the hospital's front entrance. "Sophia, I know you're busy. Why please have a Nursing Assistant take me or better yet, since I don't have any belongings, let my sister transport me," I pleaded. "No, it will be my pleasure," she politely insisted.

I told Ellen not to bother with clothing for the ride home, especially since Sophia had already given me a clean second hospital gown to wear backward like a robe to keep my derriere covered. Sporting the pair of slip-on tennis shoes Ellen brought me, I felt fully prepared for the ride home on that unseasonably warm early October evening.

My first challenge was getting into the car, especially since my arms were currently unavailable to provide any assistance whatsoever. As if sensing my concern, Ellen and Sophia both stopped talking and stared while I backed up, sat down slowly, and swung my legs into the vehicle. First challenge down. Sophia gave another warm goodbye while Ellen buckled my seat belt.

Home, James, or in this case, home...Ellen.

When we pulled into the driveway, I noticed not just one neighbor, but the entire neighborhood was out in full force, enjoying the nice weather. Even though they were uncharacteristically unavailable in the moments following the accident, I was glad they were visible now in a display of comforting normalcy.

Bob, the next-door neighbor, looked over and called out, "Hey, what happened to you?" "It's a long story. Stop over later," I called back and waited for Ellen to unlock the door so that I could take my first step back into the comfort and safety of my own home.

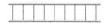

Just as I had assured the Residents, a bevy of family and friends provided me with a tremendous amount of social, emotional, and physical support from the moment I returned home. I was glad Ellen was a frequent visitor, as she was a thread I could trace back to the moments just after the accident. More than anyone, she understood what I had been through, and her support meant so much.

True to his word, Bill pulled in the driveway shortly after our arrival. By the time he walked into the living room, I was already in my recliner with both arms propped up on pillows. His presence and jovial manner filled the room, but one look at me and his face clouded with concern. "What happened? This is crazy!" After briefly recounting my ill-fated attempt at home improvement, he reminded me, "…you know tools aren't your thing. Stick to teaching!" and then sat down, waiting for a response.

I believe I surprised him when I offered no push-back whatsoever. Instead, I said only, "you're right. I won't do it again. I'm not very good at tools. Never have been. I'll have my brother come by and take what he wants. Maybe just leave me with a hammer, screwdriver…you know…a small sensible homeowner's toolbox."

A comfortable silence followed after we decided I was lucky to be alive, home from the hospital, and on the road to recovery. Three Days in Safety. Not much of a track record yet, but each day would add another to the total.

I dozed off and woke to the sound of Bill and my sister in the kitchen laughing and fixing a snack. I sat down at the table and awkwardly tried to feed myself. "Do you want help?" Ellen asked, and I said rather firmly, "No. Let me try to do it myself." Studying the plate in front of me, I took a plastic fork and somehow inserted it carefully under the wrapping on my left hand. It didn't hurt, and I didn't see any harm in doing that, especially after I successfully, yet clumsily, managed to get some food into my mouth.

"Ok, good for you," Ellen said, nodding with approval.

"Sometimes, it's the little things. I will never take anything for granted again."

A bit later, as I prepared for bedtime, I used the same method to insert my toothbrush under the same wrap on the left hand and successfully brushed my teeth. Not perfect, but this experience didn't require perfect, just survival. I selected clothes for the next day using 'ability to don with minimal/no help' as the only criteria. I found a few oversized t-shirts and two pairs of pull-up shorts and felt quite empowered when I dressed the following day independently.

Over breakfast, Bill asked me about the surgical repair of my right arm.

The surgery! Things were going so well I had almost forgotten about it.

"Well, it's scheduled for tomorrow at 1 pm. We'll leave the house at 10:30 am just to be on the safe side. I'm trying not to think about it too much. I can't have anything to eat or drink after midnight. In the meantime, let's eat!"

The rest of the day was somber, as I knew what was to follow tomorrow. I slept fitfully that night but woke surprisingly optimistic. The surgical repair to my right arm would be a painful yet vital step in my recovery, and I felt quite future-oriented when we left for the hospital.

CHAPTER 13

SURGERY (AKA "THE UNDERWEAR CAPER")

*The ritual of making patients coming to the oper-
ating theatre and remove their underwear is the
"most illogical of rituals."*
Brown

AS OPPOSED TO the solemn trip to the hospital the week before, this outing was more upbeat,
especially with Bill in the car. His sense of humor
and relaxed demeanor would put anyone at ease, and I
often told him he should have been a Nurse. He shrugs
off the compliment, but after seeing him in action since
my discharge from the hospital, I told him he had been
drafted as an honorary Nurse, and there was nothing he

could do about it. I was also glad he was there to keep Ellen engaged and distracted. This time she wouldn't wait alone, and that meant a lot to me.

My feet felt very heavy as we walked in the shadows of the hospital's central tower and toward the Outpatient Surgery Center. Nevertheless, I knew this trip was necessary, and at least I wasn't going to be admitted again. After a brief wait, I registered with the clerk, a young female employee who never identified herself called me back and abruptly asked me to remove all of my clothing and place it in a locker.

"Everything?"

"Everything"

"Even my underwear?"

"Yes, even your underwear," the highly assertive yet unidentified employee replied quite matter-of-factly. When I asked her why I had to remove my underwear for a surgical repair of my right arm, she smiled as though she was patting a child on the head and said, "Because that's the rule."

"I know, but can you please tell me why? I'd rather not expose myself..."

"Ask one of the Nurses, sir!" she replied tersely and, with a shrug, turned and left. I put my clothing in a locker and gave the key to Ellen. I sat down perplexed, waiting for someone to provide me with a cogent, logical reason why I had to remove my underwear for an outpatient planned surgery involving another part of my body.

The wait to be called back to the holding area seemed awkward and interminable. Although Ellen and Bill were with me, there wasn't much dialogue. What was there to discuss? I was going to leave them very soon to have a painful, invasive procedure, yet another bit of tangible evidence that something terrible had happened in my world.

After a wait of nearly an hour, a female voice called out "Foley," and, after quick good-byes, I was ushered to the holding area where two Nurses converged on me at once. One started the IV while the other asked me many questions about any previous experiences with anesthesia. I wondered if the man standing with them was the anesthesiologist, but on inspection of his name tag, I noted he was a CRNA (Certified Registered Nurse Anesthetist). The credentials were a welcomed sight, as several of my former students had gone on to pursue their CRNAs. I had written letters of recommendation for a number of them, and they kept me updated about the rigorous nature of their course of study and how their careers were progressing. Most of these former students said they felt incredibly well-prepared by their programs and felt they were making a real impact in operating rooms in our metropolitan area. *How wonderful, I thought. Nurses are bringing the art and science of our profession to the intimidating, scary OR.*

I stopped for a moment to learn this CRNAs name was Chris and then jumped right in. "Chris, I had surgery here 19 years ago and had a problem with laryngeal edema for the first 24 hours following. I felt like I was gagging and had a lot of trouble breathing. Do you have to use an ET (endotracheal tube) on me?" He looked intently at me for a just moment while I continued, "Chris, I'm a Nurse myself, and I'm just curious. The last time was really terrifying. I woke up in the PACU and could hardly breathe. They had trouble keeping my 'sats' up (oxygen saturation), and I think they had to give me a steroid to decrease the swelling, but I'm not sure." Chris gave me his full attention as I spoke. "I think I'll use an LMA. It's less invasive and hopefully won't give you as many problems after your surgery."

"LMA? I think I heard of that a long time ago, but can you refresh my memory?"

"An LMA is a laryngeal mask airway, and it won't cause as much swelling. Please don't worry. I'll be there with you and make sure you are ok. You're in good hands." Chris CRNA had the undefinable quality of authenticity, and I believed him. His presence, mindfulness, eye contact, and willingness to listen put me at ease.

Now, if someone would just put Chris CRNA in charge of the underwear policy, I might get an answer to my question…

Another presence suddenly filled the room, and I was face-to-face with the ubiquitous Plastics Hand Surgeon who would perform my surgery. As opposed to Chris CRNA's mindful attentiveness, this Surgeon seemed rushed and was thus brief and to the point, telling me that once the metal plate was inserted in my wrist, I would no longer require a bulky wrap dressing, only a removable splint. He would also remove the dressing to my left arm and see what he could do to give me more use of my left hand.

"Doctor, I know this is a teaching hospital, but I would prefer if you performed my surgery. I'm a teacher myself, but I am reluctant to have a surgical Resident perform my surgery. I watched a video online, and it seems like such a delicate procedure. I need my hands…"

"Fine. I'll do the surgery myself. Don't worry."

Are you sure, doctor? Stay just a minute longer to convince me…

Some thoughts flooded my mind as he turned and left quite abruptly. *"Snob! Hypocrite! You are a teacher, but you ask the attending—and not one of his Residents—to do the procedure when it comes to your own surgery. Some teacher you are!* I admit I almost called the Surgeon back to let him know one of his Residents *could* perform the procedure under his supervision but then decided to let it go. *"You've got enough to worry about. Just have the Attending Surgeon do the procedure and sort out any feelings of guilt later…"*

Two other Nurses named Cyndi and Janet appeared at that very moment, rescuing me from my maladaptive internal dialogue. Just as I did with the two younger Nurses in the ER's holding area the week before, I quickly struck up a conversation with Cyndi, an older Nurse who happened to be an alumnus of the school where I was currently teaching. She eagerly shared her goal of returning to graduate studies and asked lots of questions ranging from the program's cost to specific instructor's teaching styles. "Is Mrs. X---- still there?" interjecting "I *hope* not!" before I could answer.

Awkward!

Apparently, Mrs. X, who Cyndi described as "just not very nice," was at the epicenter of Cyndi's tragic nursing school narrative. Like the rest of us, she must have had a challenging experience in her pre-licensure program and said she didn't want to return to graduate studies if the faculty in our Master's Degree in Nursing Program were at all similar to Mrs. X. I assured her my colleagues *were* nice but would also expect her to work hard.

"That's ok," she replied. "I can handle working hard as long as they treat me good. So, what types of MSNs do you offer? I think I might want to go into teaching. Do you have an MSN focusing on education?" She continued to ask questions even as I was being wheeled down the hall to the OR suite. Jane just stood by smiling pleasantly during the entire exchange and squeezed my shoulder as I left the pre-op area. What an excellent way to distract me as I prepared for surgery by grounding me in a discussion on teaching, a topic I knew so well. I later felt vindicated to learn Cyndi enrolled in a local MSN Program within a few months of our conversation. Nevertheless, she selected another program where she determined the faculty were indeed 'nicer.' God bless her!

Now at the operating room's entrance, I was suddenly quite terrified. Supine, the bright lights above seemed to hypnotize me as I tried to convince myself this wasn't happening to me. A noticeable change in temperature and a distinct medicinal smell let me know the operating room was just beyond the next door. Once inside, I turned to see two Nurses standing over me in scrubs and disposable bouffant caps. "Hi David," one of them called out. "We're going to have you scoot over onto the table, ok?"

"Sure," but I hope the cart is locked. I have enough broken bones already." Both Nurses laughed out loud, and one of them said, "Yes, trust us, we've been doing this for a long time. It's all good."

I wanted to say something more about accident prevention, something like it only takes one slip for a severe accident to occur, but refrained. This simply wasn't the time nor the place. Be 'wholly compensatory' and keep me safe while I reside at the bottom of Maslow's Hierarchy of Needs, hoping just to wake up alive and begin the process of healing. Just take good care of me....*please.*

I was relieved when Chris CRNA, my new nursing hero, walked into the room. "David, please take a few deep breaths of this fresh air," one of the OR Nurses soothed. "Fresh air, huh? Liar!" I called back, and we all laughed again. I guess if you have to have surgery to have a metal plate inserted into your wrist to repair broken bones, sharing a light-hearted moment with the OR staff is a good thing.

And as this doctorally-prepared Nurse educator and a firm believer in evidence-based practice drifted off to sleep, I stuck out my tongue almost imperceptibly hoped no one noticed.

I still had my underwear on...

Quite proud of my defiance, a hint of a smile formed on my face as the room quickly faded to black.

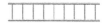

I remembered nothing more until a very pretty younger Nurse tapped my chin and said, "Take some deep breaths, David. Come on now…" I breathed as deeply as I could, feeling the fullness of a nasal cannula against my nostrils. When I had surgery nearly 20 years earlier, the post-op Nurses had a hard time keeping the oxygen level in my blood up to a safe level, so one of them elevated the bed and stood next to me, calling for me to breathe. As I suspected, my Surgeon later confirmed I had laryngeal edema (swelling in my throat) more than likely due to having a relatively narrow windpipe, a congenital defect. The experience of gasping for air was so terrifying. I was relieved not to be experiencing it again. Thanks to CRNA Chris and his LMA, I was amazed at how freely I could take in deep breaths. Sure enough, I woke sometime later to see Chris CRNA standing next to me. "How are you doing, David?" he asked. "I'm doing much better than last time. My breathing's OK, and I don't feel any swelling at all. Thank you so much!" "I'm glad to hear that. If you need anything, let us know," and he left. *How amazing he stopped by to check on me. A total class act….*

Although I never learned her name, the Post Anesthesia Care Unit (PACU) Nurse was polite and highly efficient, moving back and forth between me and another patient, who was mysteriously sequestered behind the curtain to my left. She spent most of her time with the other patient, and I heard equipment being moved around. I didn't know, nor needed to know, but of course, the nosy Nurse in me *wanted* to know. Still very drowsy, I thought, *"What did Monte Hall used to say on Let's Make a Deal? Behind curtain number one, we have…."* I just looked up at the ceiling and focused.

Mind your own business and just breathe.

I really disliked being in a post-anesthesia haze. I felt so groggy as I drifted in and out of sleep but was pleasantly surprised by how little pain I felt. I really wanted to be more alert, sensing there was so much to see and experience in the PACU, but ultimately just leaned deeply into the stupor and slept.

I opened my eyes to see Ellen and Bill standing on either side of the cart peering down at me. I could tell from their faces it had been a long wait. From prior experience working in the hospital's Pre-Surgical Testing Department, I knew that surgery cases starting in the afternoons usually run behind. *I surmised that if you're going to have surgery and are the least bit worried about time, have it first thing in the morning; otherwise, you inherit the challenges of operational delays like short staffing, urgent cases, and equipment/supply needs.* No one had told them my surgery began almost two hours late, and so they had endured a long anxious wait.

Curiously, a staff member in the waiting room offered them a pager so they could feel free to leave the crowded, noisy surgery waiting room area. Magazines and coffee in hand, they chose to flee to the more controlled chaos of the cafeteria. After waiting for two hours, they returned to the surgical waiting room to inspect an electronic screen displaying patients' first names and updates on their progress. A name displayed on the board in yellow indicated the patient was still in the pre-op area. The color changed to orange when the patient went into the OR and to green another as soon as they reached the Post-Anesthesia Care Unit (PACU). As with most systems, the output is only as timely and accurate as that entered by staff, a polite way of saying 'garbage in, garbage out.' Later, Ellen and Bill told me my color on the board never changed from yellow, and they were frankly too bashful to approach the clerk. Instead, they both experienced a very long wait with no updates. Despite the post-anesthesia haze, I could tell my sister was not too happy. "What time was it?" I asked her. "9," she replied

9 PM? Are you kidding me?

I last saw them just before 1 pm and was advised the surgery would take approximately two hours. They looked tired and hungry but were polite enough not to complain. They later said they weren't worried about waiting but instead wondered if something had happened to me. They asked the Surgical Waiting Room's clerk twice but were told they would know something as soon as *she* knew something, which never happened. After another hour, they contemplated asking her again, but she caught their gaze across the waiting room and silenced them with 'a look.'

"Excuse me (miss politely super-efficient-no -one-needs-to-know-my-name-because-I'm busy -keeping-people-alive PACU Nurse)," I called out. Her face peeped around the curtain, and I asked how soon I could leave. My family had been waiting so long...

"I'll get you out of here just as soon as I can. We're helping someone over here." In the meantime, a Nurse Technician gave me some juice and crackers and helped me transfer to a chair. About 20 minutes later, another Nurse, also cloaked in anonymity, appeared to announce she was doing my discharge.

"Ok, I can stand, transfer, eat, and drink," I thought, *"but please don't ask me to urinate. I can do that at home. Please."* It was my understanding that after outpatient surgery, the nursing staff will ask the patient to urinate before discharge. Luckily, this Nurse did not insist. Instead, she told me to be sure to 'pee' when I returned home and call if I hadn't done so within 8 hours. She also provided recommendations for my diet, a follow-up appointment, and a prescription for pain medication.

I changed back into my clothes, and we left. The cool early October evening's air was a welcomed relief as we exited the hospital and approached the car. I asked Ellen and Bill if they wanted to stop and get a bite on the way home, and they both laughed. "No," my sister replied, "We're taking you right home, and then *I'm* going home."

That's fine, Ellen, you have more than done your duty...twice

I briefly related my 'underwear' story, and at least we were all laughing as the car left the parking lot.

Take everything off indeed...

CHAPTER 14

OUR LADY OF PERPETUAL PAIN RELIEF

Never believe that a few caring people can't change
the world. For, indeed, that's all who ever have.
Margaret Mead

THE QUIET DRIVE home involved a quick trip
through a local pharmacy to fill a prescription for my
pain medication. *More narcotics. I don't want them.
I think I overheard one of the Nurses say the Surgeon usually injects a long-acting narcotic into the surgical site, so I
assumed it would be acceptable to wait until tomorrow to
have the prescription filled. I just wanted to go home and
sleep…but no…both Ellen and Bill insisted our route would*

take us right past the pharmacy, and we would have them filled now. After all, I might need them later.

It turned out they were absolutely right.

Two hours later, Ellen had gone home, Bill was in the kitchen fixing himself a late-night snack, and I was laying in the recliner watching TV with all three cats in snuggly attendance. During a commercial, I glanced down at my right hand and forearm, now encased only in a removable splint, thanks to a metal plate and many titanium screws.

The sedate, comfortable late evening's milieu abruptly changed as I called out in sudden pain, and Bill, sandwich in hand, came running. I'm sure he was shocked to see me in such a state of sudden and incredible discomfort, especially since I had just told him I was doing fine a few minutes earlier. As he stood there looking at me with a quizzical expression, any last whisperings of the general sedation and the long-acting narcotic injection worn off in unison. Incapable of speech, I could only respond to his questions with the same guttural "ahhs" I had emitted during the moments after the accident. A few minutes later, Bill, now really concerned, asked if he should call 911. I put my left arm up in a halting gesture and said, "Wait." After some deep breathing and repositioning, some coherent thoughts returned, and I announced the honeymoon was over—it was now time to do battle with terrible post-op incisional and bone pain resulting from multiple screws inserted into my arm.

"Bring me those pain pills." *Thank God we had the prescription filled...*

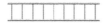

"Although we should take all pain seriously, bone pain and pleuritic (lung) pain are among the worst types of pain," was a point frequently made by a number of my nursing instructors. I passed the same message along to many of my students, especially as they reflected on patients who were rude, profane, or simply outright mean. "Please be understanding, as your patients may not exactly be themselves while they experience excruciating discomfort. Do what you can for them and be empathetic, even if they are very unpleasant."

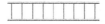

Despite the pain, I had no plans of being rude to *anyone*, especially in my own living room. All I wanted was some relief! As my groans intensified, my three cats scurried off the recliner and stood staring at me from various parts of the room.

In a rapid, pressured speech, I told Bill it felt like the effects of the anesthesia had dissipated just as though someone had turned on a light switch. I was lying there watching TV in a state of relative comfort one moment and BOOM...literally out of my mind with pain the next. I was concerned, as there must be a serious reason for such rapid onset. Visions of terrible post-surgical complications danced in front of me: a blood clot? Fatty embolus? Did one of the screws pierce a nerve? Any of these complications was potentially debilitating at the least and life-threatening at the worst. *Oh no...a serious post-surgical complication resulting in an adverse outcome—or death—within 24 hours after surgery. A sentinel event with a root cause analysis...this time about me...How many days in safety am I?*

"I can't take this, I can't TAKE THIS, I CAN'T TAKE THIS!!!!!" I screamed without waiting for him to ask any more questions. "Take what? WHAT IS THE MATTER WITH YOU???" he asked me as I curled up into a ball and screamed, "Pain! Ugggghhh! HELP ME!!!!" The cats had finally had enough and scampered downstairs as he handed me the pills and a small glass of water. The pain was so intense I just wanted it to end as quickly as possible. Frankly, I was tempted to take more than the prescribed dose but reasoned that since I am highly susceptible to narcotics, I would feel the effects of just the prescribed dose very quickly.

In the meantime, Bill sat down and stared at me in disbelief. "Calm down and tell me what's is going on!" I offered no reply but asked him to turn off the TV and shut off a nearby lamp as even the noise and the light hurt. I rocked back and forth with my eyes closed, waiting for the narcotics to attack the pain, my new unwelcomed adversary. *But you usually have a very high tolerance for pain...took nothing other than Acetaminophen after your gall bladder surgery and never bothered to have the prescription filled after that dental procedure...*

"You were doing so well," Bill interrupted my thoughts. "What can I do?"

"Nothing," I interrupted. "Just please don't leave. Please sit there just in case...."

"OK, I got it...I'm right here." Bill finished his snack and dozed off.

An hour later, the pain was even worse. "Bill! Something's wrong! I may have to go back to the Emergency Room. This is not normal! It's worse than right after the accident! Oh no..." Snapped to attention by my cries, even Bill, the congenial diplomat, had had enough. He walked over and looked intently at my hand. "Nothing's wrong. I'm not a Nurse but look at your hand. It's pink and warm. Swollen, but that's understandable, and it looks ok." He held up my discharge instructions, saying, "It's late, but do you think we should call the 'Nurse Advice Line' listed on this paper?"

Call the Nurse Advice Line? Just let me think for a second....

SHARON!!!!!!!!

My trusted colleague...the Queen of Pharmacology from the School of Nursing! We collaborated well on many projects, and she gave me much-needed advice as I proceeded through the dissertation process. As a colleague, clinician, and friend, I trusted her opinion completely. "I'll gladly call the best Nurse Advice Line I know right now. Can you help me dial this number?"

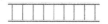

223

2001

I was in the middle of a 12-week temporary agency contract working in an ICU at a local hospital. The hospital's full-time Nurses seemed to look down on us 'temporaries,' as there was an apparent assumption we were only 'in it for the money' and weren't interested in providing safe, quality care. One day a 'regular' Nurse came by and issued a stern warning: "you better make sure you have all your T's crossed, and I's dotted because the Nurse who's following you is just excellent and demands nothing less than total perfection...."

Oh yeah?

Never one to shirk from a challenge, I made sure I had 'taken off' all Physician orders, given all medications, charted thoroughly, and took special care that each patient was presentable and their rooms clean. When change-of-shift arrived, I made a few final notes and looked up to see a rather unassuming female standing next to me. "Are you following me," I asked? She nodded, and with no pleasantries whatsoever, I gave the most thorough report I had ever provided to an oncoming Nurse (I even insisted on walking her through the patients' rooms to make sure all was in good order). Before I left, I wrote down my phone number and said, "Now, if you have any questions about my care, charting, or anything at all, please call me, even if it's in the middle of the night. I take pride in my work and would rather hear any complaints from you directly rather than someone else."

Looking at me quizzically, she said, "Oh, I'm sure everything will be ok, and by the way, my name is Sharon…." For a moment, I was just a bit embarrassed. I was so intent on giving her a thorough report that I hadn't even introduced myself.

I went home, slept soundly, and never heard from her. When I reported back for work the next day, she followed me again, and I gave her nursing report on the same two patients and left. I felt quite vindicated when I heard a colleague whisper that Sharon had been uncharacteristically quiet. In my mind, that meant things must have gone well, and I left with a smile. Although I did not cross paths with Sharon—the Nurse with the incredibly high standards—again at that hospital, she left a deep impression on me.

Although I was initially affronted, I ultimately chose to rise to the challenge. All nurses—not just Sharon—following me should get the same thorough report and attention to detail. I took note of that lesson very carefully. Rather than becoming adversarial with Sharon and other Nurses like her, I vowed to work harder to meet their standards, and in doing so, my own standard was enhanced. In fact, it wasn't too long until I realized other Nurses might say I, too, was a Sharon. In any case, that singular encounter had a profound impact on my nursing practice and gave me an interesting anecdote to share with students as they prepared to enter professional nursing practice. The message was loud and clear: keep the focus on quality patient care and leave personalities out of it.

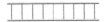

2012

Two weeks before my first day as a full-time instructor at a local school of nursing, I received an email from one of the nursing faculty offering lots of advice along with a kind offer to help acclimate me to the University's complex, highly political environment.

The email was signed, "Most sincerely….Sharon."

On the first day, I entered the office suite and was amazed to see Sharon was the "cross your T's and dot your I's" Nurse from so many years ago. Incredibly, Sharon remembered meeting me and even recalled me offering her my phone number. "You were so nervous…"

No, I was not nervous. Just determined.

"Well, I had a right to be," I retorted! "You had quite the reputation as a prima donna!" We both laughed, and I was relieved that I knew at least one person at the University. We went to lunch that day and talked for three hours, setting the stage for a long and productive friendship. Sharon and I shared so much over the next few years. Although we collaborated on multiple projects related to teaching, she also helped me shape my nursing identity and teaching philosophy.

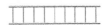

Since I now counted her among my closest friends, I doubted she would mind if I called her, even it meant waking her up. It was unforgivably late, but I needed advice. She taught the Pharmacology courses in each of the pre-licensure nursing programs, and I knew she could help me figure out how to relieve this terrible pain. As a veritable encyclopedia of nursing knowledge, she would know exactly what to do.

Bill took my cell phone, found her number on my contacts list, and handed me the phone when it started ringing. It rolled to voice mail, so I called again and was so relieved when she answered sleepily.

"Sharon, I'm so very sorry to call this late," my voice sounded forcibly calm and very odd, perhaps in the same carefully restrained and unnatural tone and cadence as when I called Ellen on the day of the accident. "I had surgery today, and I can't take the pain. Please help me! I took narcotics, but it didn't work. My hand is pink and warm, so I think the surgery went ok and it's not a matter of poor circulation. I can move my fingers, but they're still pretty swollen... I just can't take the pain anymore. Help me please! Sharon..."

"Do you have any Ibuprofen in the house," Sharon asked? "If so, take some of that. The nerve endings in your bones are all aggravated from the surgery, and I bet that would help to decrease the swelling and inflammation and calm them down. Take some Acetaminophen too. It's ok to take them together because they work differently. Be sure to take another round of narcotics as soon as it's time. That should get you through until morning but call me back if you need to."

Ibuprofen, Tylenol, and narcotics? Really?

"Sharon, are you sure it's ok to take all that?" I asked, immediately feeling foolish for doing so. Sharon was a true pharmacology maven, and as one of my mentors, I respected her so much. Just as she began to answer, I interrupted, saying, "Sharon, I'm sorry…of course it's ok; otherwise, you wouldn't have told me to take them. If that doesn't work, I'll need you to come over and hit me over the head with a board, and maybe that will help." As we laughed, I became more hopeful but still acutely aware of the icy, searing pain. "Seriously though, David, that should help, but if it doesn't, call me back, and I will run over and look at your hand. I don't care what time it is."

I thanked her profusely, made a mental note to be sure to pay her kindness forward to as many people as possible, and then meekly did precisely as she instructed. I had never before stopped to consider how severe out-of-control pain can cause cognitive disorganization and was thankful Bill was there to ensure I took the proper medications in the right amounts. A bit later, I dutifully took another round of narcotics, closed my eyes, and waited.

Incredibly, no *miraculously*, within a short time the pain was not only improved but *gone,* just like that. The same intra-psychic switch that suddenly flipped 'on' and unleashed wave after wave of unbelievable pain was switched 'off,' and with that, the pain, discomfort, and cognitive disorganization were all gone. It was almost like feeling a cool, refreshing breeze that gently but firmly drove the pain far from me. I fell into a deep, nourishing sleep in the recliner and woke up 7 hours later to broad daylight. Reality flooded back, and I quickly wondered if the pain had returned, but no, it hadn't.

For the rest of that day, I felt nothing but an incredibly tolerable gentle, dull ache on movement, but if I kept my arm close to my chest, I felt nothing at all. Nothing. Just for good measure, I took a few more rounds of Ibuprofen and Acetaminophen, monitoring those doses carefully to ensure I stayed within the safe daily limits. That was it. I didn't need any more narcotics, and the bottle was soon banished to the top shelf of my medicine cabinet.

Later that afternoon, I wondered how I could possibly repay Sharon for helping me and laughed out loud when I thought of the perfect way to memorialize her kindness. I began referring to her as 'Our Lady of Perpetual Pain Relief,' which made her very happy when she called for an update on my progress.

I was so glad I had embraced Sharon as a colleague and not chose to view her as an adversary over a decade before. Perhaps some Nurses—even me—might have assumed a confrontational "who do you think you are?" or "you can't tell me what to do?" stance, but on that day, I chose to rise to meet her standards and in doing so, made a wonderful friend and colleague. I had friends, and I had *friends*. As with Bill, Sharon was a *friend* and proved that over and over as the next two months progressed. Each time I greeted her, I made a bowing motion and called her by her most reverend new name as she laughed heartily.

Unfortunately for me, two days later, Bill told me he would have to return to Detroit but promised to return once again if I needed him. Need him? I dreaded being alone in this compromised state where even the most mundane tasks took so much longer than usual. Later that morning, when Bill was in the shower, I tried to pour myself a cup of coffee and carry it to the living room. I managed to *pour* the coffee but sadly introduced it to the living room floor only a minute later. What would I do when he left?

Bill made sure he went to the grocery store and stocked me with a variety of finger-food items and even thought to open several pull-top cat food cans and cover them with snap-on lids that I could open. Even the cats benefitted from his kindness. He cleaned the cat boxes, straightened up the house, and said goodbye. God bless him.

He closed the front door and was gone, leaving me alone for the first time since the accident. Ironically, I found myself standing in the same spot where I placed the distress call to my sister. I watched his shiny maroon Ford 500 disappear as he left the development and felt silence envelop me.

Besides my immediate family, Bill and Sharon were the two best examples of what Dr. Betty Neuman, my nursing hero, would call integral parts of my 'lines of defense.' Ellen, Bill, and Sharon certainly did help me re-establish some sense of security and control in my life. Without them, I don't know what I would have done, and was awash with gratitude for their help. At the same time, however, I was confronted with the sobering thought of the number of people who lacked an Ellen, Bill, or Sharon in their life. How would they have coped with a similar injury and recover?

The best I could do for now was vow to be an Ellen, Bill, or Sharon to other friends or loved ones in the future and focus on preparing for the challenges of the weeks ahead.

PART VI

THERE'S SAFETY IN NUMBERS

CHAPTER 15

STUDENTS AND FAMILY TO THE RESCUE

"...Love your neighbor as yourself."
Matthew 22:39

SHORTLY AFTER BILL left, I sat down at the kitchen table, already thinking about the next steps in my recovery. The first thing I did was perform an inventory of my ADLs (activities of daily living). Although I had a supportive network of family and friends, the encroaching reality of living alone quickly overcame me. I wanted to check my emails, continue working on a publication and complete a grant application, but what did I *need* to accomplish today?

- Take care of the kitties (of course, they come first)
- Feed myself
- Take a sponge bath (now that should be very interesting)
- Shave
- Call my parents and ask them to come over
- *Some gloriously ambitious agenda, Nurse Foley.*

Since Bill had already fed the cats, much to their delight, I slipped them some extra treats and then moved to the bathroom, where I found an old electric razor in a drawer. Finding it surprisingly easy to maneuver, I managed to shave quite well.

Check!

I carefully laid out my new favorite oversized t-shirt and a pair of pull-up shorts, got undressed, and filled the sink with warm water. Being very careful not to get my incision wet, I did *reasonably* well bathing myself and, after dressing, even managed to wash my hair (well, sort of…). I changed, combed my hair, and headed to the kitchen for lunch.

Check, check, check!!!

Just then, the familiar, welcomed sight of my parents' car greeted me as they pulled into the driveway. I moved to the recliner so they could see me clean, relaxed, and smiling as they entered.

See folks, now just relax. Everything's going to get back to be okay. There's no need to worry.

In true parental form, they didn't fall for my veneer of normalcy. Not one bit. My mom was teary-eyed when she sat down, and my dad, ever the Safety Team Leader, attempted to broach the elephant in the living room. "Now that the worst is behind you, will you please tell me what happened?" he asked. Audibly sighing, I asked him to step into the garage while my mom made coffee. "Would you like something to eat," she asked? "Um, ok, I guess," I called back as nonchalantly as I could manage. "Would you please make me a sandwich?" *Are you kidding, mom? I would love a 'mom' sandwich. I'm starving!*

I opened the door to the garage door and stepped inside. It was the first time I had been there since the accident, and I suddenly felt my heart quickening. "Now tell me what happened," my dad again requested as I walked around looking at the untouched scene. "Well, I was on the ladder holding the pile driver, and it collapsed. There's not much more to it than that. I had the extension ladder leaned against the wall, and my face was all the way up there, where the wall meets the ceiling. I checked to make sure the ladder's rubber feet were secure before I went up, but I guess I pushed too hard when I started drilling, and the ladder's feet shifted, causing it to slide right down this wall." Glancing around again, I noticed drops of dried blood in various sizes telling the story, dotting the floor and leaving a trail across the garage out into the driveway and then back toward the kitchen. It seemed I fared a bit better than the pile driver, whose plastic hull lay in pieces scattered all over the floor while its disembodied lithium battery lay 15 feet away.

I could hardly look at him. We both knew there were many things I could have done that would have prevented or at least mitigated the accident. I could have asked for help by having someone hold the ladder or called my car into duty by moving it into the garage and place a board across one of the tires to brace the ladder. Better yet, I should have asked a professional to install the brackets for me and avoided the ladder altogether. "Using power tools just isn't your gift," I could hear him say. "Hire someone who knows what they are doing,"

Oh well.

At any rate, we just stood there and looked around in silence for quite some time at the spot where my delightful narrative entitled "Thousands of Days in Safety" abruptly ended. I stared intently at the wall itself, paying particular attention to the path the ladder took during its sudden plunge. Contained within that neat trajectory were some stray nails sticking out of the wall that I'm sure were used over the years to hang some long-forgotten item. I also spotted a surface-mounted electrical outlet and some sharp gardening tools near the ladder's base. I could have hit my head or snagged a body part on any one of them. As we stood staring, the true unspoken message between us was that my narrative could have ended *altogether*. "Thousands of Days in Safety...followed by an abrupt end." Instead, battered and broken, I was still alive and awash with gratitude in a new narrative called 'Ten Days (and Counting...) in Safety'.

"You're lucky," he said, and as he had done so many times during my childhood, said nothing more and simply walked stoically back into the house.

Oh yes, I agree entirely. Lucky, oh so lucky.

Admittedly trying to change the subject just a bit, I asked, "What will I use to deal with those blood-stains?" "I don't know about that. Go ask your mother," he replied, but I never did. Those bloodstains, long-faded, are still inside that garage in silent testimony to the importance of family, love, support, and…safety.

While we were outside, my mom indeed made delicious 'mom' sandwiches to add to the fresh fruit and side dishes she had brought with her, and I noted the happiness in her eyes when I proceeded to eat everything in sight. After that, I asked my parents, siblings, and friends to stop by often, not just because of the food, but I surmised if nothing else, this accident presented a fantastic opportunity for us to all spend some time together.

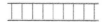

The next afternoon I heard a soft, tentative knock on the front door and was very startled to see Rebecca and Lisa, a current and former student, respectively, standing there smiling. "Ladies!" I exclaimed. "What a wonderful surprise! How did you find my address?"

"A little bird told us," Rebecca soothed as she and Lisa entered, each carrying a bag of supplies. As I closed the door, I noticed a large blue cooler just outside the front door, and they confirmed they had it placed there. "What for?" I asked. "Well, your current and former students have decided to help you during your time of need," Lisa offered, "Please don't object."

Ladies, it's nice of you to stop by, but what is this?

Reading my mind, Rebecca continued, "We put together an online 'Care Calendar' with spots for people to sign up to bring you meals, provide help around the house, lawn care, rides to appointments, errands… anything you need."

"Oh ladies, that's very generous of you, but I just can't."

Lisa jumped in, saying, "Oh yes, you can, Dr. Foley. We arranged the whole thing, and a bunch of people have already responded. You helped us. Now it's time for us to help *you*. We've taken care of everything! After all, you didn't nickname us the 'Dynamic Duo' for nothing!"

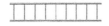

Spring Semester 2015

On the first day of Nursing 100, I gazed out into the audience, and one student really stood out. I guessed we were about the same age as she stared at me with an intensity that conveyed a combination of self-doubt and terror. Over the next two hours, my gaze fixed on her several times, and I almost called on her but instinctively held back. I wasn't surprised when she came up to the podium immediately after class to introduce herself. "Hello, my name is Lisa, and I don't think I can do this. Do you have any advice for me?" I asked her to step into my office, and she immediately launched into a well-ingrained narrative of self-doubt. She had already raised her family and was returning to school to pursue a career in nursing but doubted she could handle the pressure.

"I don't know how to study, and I know *absolutely nothing* about computers! What am I going to do?" After calming her down for a few minutes, I offered the usual 'how to succeed in your first semester of nursing school' advice: be sure to read, stay organized, practice in the skills lab, find a study partner (or group), and whatever you do, don't procrastinate!

We parted ways, and over the next few weeks, I noticed her intently taking notes in my class. She did well on the first exam, and I observed with relief that her Nurse Theorist paper, worth 30 percent of the course's grade, was outstanding. Because of these hard-won victories, I was shocked to see her crying outside the School of Nursing's administrative offices a few weeks later.

"Lisa, what's wrong?"

"I just can't do this. I don't think I will ever be able to do this," she replied weakly. We sat down on a nearby bench as she sobbed, "I'm just barely passing Pathophysiology, and I'm not sure my clinical instructor likes me."

"Lisa, this is your first semester, and this is all new to you, especially at...well...*our* age. Just like you, I returned to school after a long time away, and it's been a huge adjustment for me too. Just remember, getting a 'C' in nursing school doesn't mean failure. It means 'continue,' and you're going to do just that—continue! Just keep showing up for clinicals, turn in your assignments, and ask your clinical instructor for some feedback. Maybe it's not as bad as you think. You can do this, Lisa! Get yourself organized, study, and do well on your Patho test! I glanced down and saw a 'Go-Gos' sticker on her book. "Lisa, no way! The Go-Gos are one of my all-time favorite groups! Come on now, remember they had the beat…now *you* got the beat! It's your turn. Go home and get to work. This first semester is almost over, and the next will be better. If nothing else, at least you'll know what to expect." We parted laughing, and I said a silent prayer for her success.

Amid the hubbub end-of-semester wrap-up activities, I lost track of her. I was delighted, however, when she returned to school the next semester and was so proud to inform me that she had passed all her classes. "Just remember, Lisa, the material might be more complex, but from here on out, it's more of the same: reading, lectures, exams, skills lab test-outs, case studies, clinicals, and care plans. At least you will know what to expect."

Over the next year, Lisa participated in some school of nursing activities, and it was such a pleasure to watch her tentativeness morph into a carefully restrained form of confidence. At 'pinning,' the private, hallowed cere-mony that takes place just before commencement, I must admit I was teary-eyed when Lisa was handed her pin. Afterward, I assured her that much good would result from her experiences in the program. I perceived her to be a role model for 'non-traditional' students returning to school, and I hoped she would return as an alumnus to inspire others.

Only time would tell.

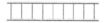

Spring Semester 2016

On the day of Nursing 100, I again looked out into the audience and saw two 'non-traditional' students, both female, sitting in the front row listening intently to my lectures. One of these students, Rebecca, took great pride in her note-taking, and together with her seatmate, developed a set of beautifully color-coded notes. When I spoke with Rebecca, she appeared very confident and polished, although I still detected some self-doubt. She had many questions about the program in general and wondered if there were any former students from whom she could solicit some much-needed advice.

Lisa!!!

Well into the dissertation process, I recalled the concept of social capital and recognized how powerful it would be to introduce Rebecca and Lisa. I contacted Lisa, and she readily agreed to a meeting. Two weeks later, Rebecca enthusiastically reported that she and Lisa met, talked, and became fast friends. Like Lisa, Rebecca was working hard to maintain a school-life balance. As time moved forward, it seemed Rebecca and Lisa complemented each other very well. Lisa provided Rebecca with many tips and 'insider social capital.' At the same time, Rebecca seemed to inspire Lisa with just a bit more self-confidence as she passed the NCLEX-RN and moved forward into professional nursing practice.

It appeared to be a match made in heaven. In fact, I dubbed them a 'Dynamic Duo.' Seeing their friendship blossom, I continued to use what I called the 'power of the podium' to introduce other students to each other and, in essence, help them augment their social capital too. I sometimes heard the all-too-familiar tale of "I'm the first person in my family to go to college, and I feel lost" or acted on instinct when I approached a student sitting by themselves, appearing isolated and alone. In any case, I played 'yenta' and introduced alumni to current students, seniors to sophomores, sophomores to juniors, etc. I was meticulous about asking students permission before making such connections, but they almost always said yes.

This 'yenta-ing' was so successful that in her senior year, I asked Rebecca to help me with the "Minority Association of Nursing Students (MANS)," for which I served as faculty advisor. Together we came up with the idea of creating a mentoring program for students and invited them to a "Red Carpet" event at the beginning of the fall semester. The event's theme was "MANS Starring…YOU!" and as the students walked the carpet, we encouraged them to have their pictures taken before they entered a room filled with students from all levels in the nursing program, alumni, and of course, faculty. Our collective message, loud and clear, was "there's no need to be alone." The students were so enthusiastic in their response, so we vowed to have another such event the next month.

Unfortunately, the accident occurred less than a week later.

Nevertheless, Rebecca continued to demonstrate authentic leadership and kept MANS moving forward until I returned. As a result of her efforts, at the end of the academic year, the School of Nursing was awarded the University's coveted "President's Award for Excellence in Diversity" for an unprecedented third year in a row.

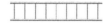

October 2016 (11 Days in Safety)

Lisa's and Rebecca's friendship was flourishing as they sat in my living room to share their kind offers of assistance. I slipped into the bedroom and placed a discrete call to the School of Nursing's Associate Dean, informing her of the student's intentions and asking her if she thought such an arrangement would be appropriate. "Absolutely," she said unflinchingly. "I think it's very sweet of them to do that," and with that validation, I listened to their plans with interest. When they left about an hour later, I offered a long prayer of thanks for having such wonderful, caring people as integral parts of my lines of defense.

Lucky, oh so lucky.

CHAPTER 16

RECONSTITUTION

*The term reconstitution in the Neuman Model of
Systems refers to the recovery of the system from
stressors (adversity) and the return to a state of
equilibrium or well being*
Sally Hannoodee and Amit S. Dhamoon

TWO DAYS LATER, I saw the welcomed site of Bill's Ford 500 pulling back into my driveway. My parents happened to be visiting when he arrived, and they were also happy to see him. Over the years, they have adopted him as an unofficial son; actually, I believe it was he who adopted *them*. In any case, he is now a welcomed addition to our family.

I hadn't been out of the house in several days. I told Bill I had an appointment at the Orthopedic Clinic to have a permanent or traditional cast, applied to my left arm, and begin occupational Therapy. Surgery behind me, I was ready to aggressively start the Reconstitution process, loosely defined within the context of the Neuman Systems Model as returning to a level of stability following a stressor.

The instructions following surgery were quite vague, leaving me unsure of my limitations. I knew the breaks in my right arm had been repaired by a metal plate affixed with many screws and should heal well, but exactly how much could I do and when could I return to work? Could I type? Drive? Start an IV? Like so many other Nurses, I was not used to just sitting around and quietly driving myself crazy thinking about these and many other questions that made up a huge, vacuous unknown. I put up a good front when others were around but had grown tired of watching TV and just wanted to return to my daily routine. With my parents, siblings, and Bill to keep me company, the days flew by, laden with plenty of good food and laughter.

During my next trip to the hospital's outpatient pavilion, I was pensive and a bit nervous. I vowed to be a motivated patient and, in doing so, hoped the Orthopedics Team and Occupational Therapy would get me back to work very soon. When I arrived at the Orthopedic Clinic's registration desk, I was confronted by a very assertive registration clerk who tersely demanded to copy my driver's license and insurance card, after which she asked me who referred me to "their clinic."

"I'm not sure how to answer your question," I told her, "but I have the 'Select' insurance plan and received a phone call to report here today at 9 am for casting and an Occupational Therapy evaluation in follow-up to my surgery last Tuesday." I even held up my right splinted arm in an apparent attempt to impress her.

Notably *unimpressed*, she continued staring at the computer screen until she found the information she was sought. "Oh, I see. Yes, you did have surgery, and I see your referral. 'They' put it in the wrong place, but I will go ahead and register you anyway. I'll have to talk to 'them' about that..." she offered as her voice trailed off.

I stared at her lips moving but disappeared into my thoughts. *Register me anyway? Of course, you should. Have to tell 'them' about that? If you must, but I don't need to be involved in any of this drama. Can I just take a seat, please?*

As if she read my mind, she silently pointed to the waiting room, and I sat down. I'm not sure if she said anything else, and I honestly didn't care. It sounded like there were some opportunities for rapid-cycle performance improvement in their referral/registration process, a chance for solid teamwork and collaboration among peers in pursuit of customer satisfaction and patient-centered care. Fix the problems, so future customers who might be in pain or de-conditioned after surgery don't have to stand here any longer than necessary. *While you're at it, please figure out why a co-worker entered a referral in the wrong place.*

"Oh sir, I'm sorry, you also need to get your arms X-rayed first. 'They' should have told you to go directly to X-ray before you came here today.

Wonderful.

"Just go down the hall to X-ray, and they (*there's that 'they' again*) will take care of you. Be sure to come right back here afterward." Since I worked at this hospital years earlier, I already knew the way and was registered by a woman who used to work in my area and remembered me immediately. "Marcia! It's so wonderful to see you. How have you been doing?" Just as I remembered, she was polite and every so efficient. She quickly registered me and made sure my X-rays were taken promptly. She even escorted me back to the Orthopedics Clinic to wish me well and personally handed my X-rays to the matter-of-fact registration clerk. "Please take good care of my friend, ok?"

Friend? As part of my exit strategy from this hospital years earlier, I made sure relationships with co-workers and employees were in good order. I recalled having a long conversation with Marcia. She and I sparred many times over various leadership/management issues, but we left things on a very positive note in the end. I saw her at a restaurant several later, and she seemed so genuine when she said, "David, we really missed you when you left." I hoped my response was equally authentic when I assured her I missed her as well, and now here she was, helping me navigate through a tedious clinical visit.

Marcia departed with a quick hug, and a few minutes later, I heard a voice politely call my name from across the room. I stood and was greeted by a smiling middle-aged woman named Donna, who introduced herself as my Occupational Therapist. She asked me what I did for a living, and after I told her, I noted she became even more attentive and proceeded with a tighter focus. "What concerns do you have about your recovery?" she asked.

"I'm so afraid I won't be able to use fine motor skills to perform some nursing procedures. I'm not working as a direct care Nurse right now, but I might return to practice someday or, at the very least, may need to demonstrate a procedure for one of my students. Help me, please…"

"How do you think you're doing so far?" Donna asked. "Your surgery was when? Oh, I see, not too long ago…."

"Donna, I'm really worried. The distal end of my right thumb is very numb and extremely weak. I can hardly move it. Do you think there might be nerve damage…?"

"Let's not get ahead of ourselves, David. I want to do a complete assessment first, but I need to remind you your recovery can take months. You have a long road ahead of you. Are you ready to get to work?"

"Yes," was all I could reply. *Long road ahead? I want to go back to work right away, but I didn't want to tell her.* What if she advised against it? I could think of many ways to overcome any obstacles. I could get a ride to work, wear easy-on clothing, have students and co-workers open doors for me…

"David, the first thing I'm going to do is measure your angle of pronation and supination. You need to put your right arm out in front of you on the table with your hand extended and try to place your palm flat on the table and then, without moving your elbow, turn your hand so your palm faces the ceiling. Doing so requires your ulna and radius to crisscross, so you probably can't do it very well right now but let's see where you are, and then I will measure your progress as time goes on."

The pain was significant, and I was disappointed by my limited range of motion, but Donna told me it was a good start. As I tried, she quickly reached over and held my elbow firmly on the table, so my wrist and hands had to do all the work on their own. Some of the maneuvers really hurt, but she assured me the plate and screws would hold everything firmly in place. "Just don't overdo it and be patient" was her consistent message.

She reinforced the highly disappointing news that the return of full dexterity in my right thumb could take months of hard work. I was currently able to only touch the tip of my thumb to the tip of my index finger. Making contact with any of the other fingers was presently out of the question.

Donna suggested I place my right forearm flat, dangle my hand over the edge of my dining room table, and then hook my thumb through a plastic grocery bag containing a single can of tuna. The goal was to attempt mini 'thumb ups' to regain strength and, ultimately, dexterity. She retrieved a plastic bag and can of tuna from her cabinet so we could try the exercise. I was disappointed I couldn't do even one thumb-up. Not one. With great difficulty, my thumb was at least able to maintain resistance against the bag, albeit shakily so.

"Just be patient, David. Your recovery will take time, but I sense your determination, and that will help. *Just be patient, David,* I silently repeated, not mocking her, but expressing frustration at the long road ahead.

Donna handed me a sheet of exercises that had quite obviously been copied many, many times. Although blurry, I imagined the exercises were tried and true and couldn't wait to get home and get to work. "We only have one other thing to do today, and that's fitting you for your new-and-improved splint. The one they gave you in surgery is OK, but we can make one much lighter and easy to maneuver. It will also be less noticeable, which will be a plus when you go back to work.

WORK?

"Donna, can we talk about that? I really want to go back to work…."

"As soon as you leave here, you'll be going to Ortho, and you can discuss that with them. We only make recommendations for Occupational Therapy, and they will handle anything beyond that." Donna's smooth delivery didn't sound the least bit rehearsed or condescending but seemed to come from a place of experience.

Yes ma'am!

I watched as she used material from her cabinet to mold a custom splint for my right wrist and forearm, and she was right—it felt equally sturdy but much lighter than the one I received after surgery. Once I put on a long shirt sleeve, no one would hardly notice…

"OK, we're all set. Please don't forget to schedule your follow-up OT appointments at the front desk before you leave. Let me check if the doctor is ready for you or if they want you to go to the casting room first."

The question answered, Donna directed me to the Casting Room around the corner, where a tall thin man named Jack asked me to sit down so he could cast my left arm.

My left arm. Even though I had suffered an avulsion fracture in my left arm and had fractured the Triquetral bone in my left wrist, my right arm, with its new metal plate and many titanium screws, had commanded most of my attention so far. Besides being a bit weak and encased in a bulky temporary cast, my left arm hadn't given me much pain or discomfort. Nonetheless, it needed to be placed in a 'permanent' cast that would be more comfortable, less bulky, and provide a more normalized appearance just in case I returned to work soon.....

Stop it!

Jack began by asking me if I had ever been casted before, and I assured him I had not. He then told me the hospital was 'fresh out' of traditional white casting material, and I would have to pick a different color.

Huh? How could a large hospital, designated as a Level I Trauma Center, run of casting material?

He presented me with several color choices, and I chose lime green since it was the closest to the School of Nursing/University's colors. *At least I can joke with the students about it.*

I admit I was amazed by the skill Jack demonstrated as he casted my arm. He immediately put me at ease as he exercised his craft with fluid, effortless efficiency. Jack's hands flew as he simultaneously worked, clearly exuding unconscious competence as he asked about the accident and my profession. He seemed particularly interested in my experiences as an educator. I was surprised to learn he had acted as a preceptor for many Casting Technicians and gave talks to the Medical Residents during their Orthopedics rotation. Before I knew it, Jack was finished, advised me to "take it easy" on the cast until it fully dried, and sent me on my way. I was inspired by his skills performed in such a highly competent yet patient-centered manner.

The clinic's operations? Now that was a different matter entirely.

I stepped out of the Casting Room and felt utterly lost. I peeked back inside, but Jack, with his energetic spirit, was already gone. Where should I go? Donna, the Occupational Therapist, had mentioned I would also see an Orthopedic Doctor, but where? "Excuse me," I said to the first person wearing scrubs. "I was just casted, and now I think I'm supposed to see a doctor. Do you know where…?"

"No, I don't," the anonymous figure said with their back to me. "Go ask at the front desk." *OK, now that narrows it down. Where is the front desk?* I wandered down the hall of the vast clinic and came upon a small Nurses Station. Asking the same question, one of the Nurses told me I had somehow found the right place and a Doctor could see me now. She explained I would "only" see a Resident during this visit regarding my left arm and that I would see "Plastics Hand" regarding my right arm sometime next week.

Oh.

I was escorted to a non-descript exam room, and soon a Senior Resident popped in and, after examining the X-rays of my left arm, told me all looked fine. He advised I should wear my splint (*but hey, that's on my right arm, and I thought that was "Plastic Hands"' domain*) and keep my new cast clean and dry. "Please keep it covered if you shower. Otherwise, it may get ruined or stink." He firmly redirected any return-to-work questions to the Plastics Hand Service and asked me to wait until one of the Junior Residents stopped by to see me. After an interminable 45 minute wait, I had had enough and just left, somehow finding my way back to the front desk. I confirmed I had my post-surgical appointment with Plastics Hand the following week and was provided a phone number to call to schedule my Occupational Therapy appointments.

Thank you. Now get me out of here.

On the way home, I thought long and hard about the visit. Yes, I was very grateful I had insurance and access to medical care. Many people don't have that luxury. I knew the road to recovery would require a lot of hard work, but I recognized recovery was a possibility, and for many, it isn't. *More gratitude, please!* I continued to stew, however, at the inefficiency of the clinic's operations, especially from the perspective of quality improvement and patient-centered care; after all, I left out of frustration. I wondered how many other patients had also not waited to see one of their providers or, worse yet, left before being seen altogether. Quality improvement was possible for these rather tortured clinical operations, but only through tremendous teamwork and collaboration.

But I wasn't there for that. I was only there to be seen and receive care. It didn't matter that I was Nurse, a former employee, or a nursing instructor. Maybe if they had known that, I might have received more efficient care, but I honestly didn't care. My goal was to remain in the role of patient and not use any pretense of status to gain special treatment. I re-entered the intellectual space bounded by my roles as a patient, educator, and Nurse and, in doing so, gathered many valuable stories to share with students. Based on today's experiences—and other similar experiences like them—I smelled many simulations and case studies in the making and took comfort in that.

PART VII

REDEFINING SAFETY

CHAPTER 17

RETURN TO RAMPANT NORMALCY

I am beginning to learn that it is the sweet, simple things of life which are the real ones after all.
Laura Ingalls Wilder

T HE WEEK FOLLOWING my casting and baptism by fire into Occupational Therapy was an excruciating exercise in boredom. The first couple of days were tolerable as I watched TV and caught up on more movies I had missed during the all-consuming dissertation process. In doing so, I felt some small measure of satisfaction in that I had re-claimed just a bit of cultural relevance. After a few more days of reality TV and pay-per-view movies, that feeling of satisfaction evaporated into nothingness.

Thankfully I also continued to receive a stream of family, friends, and students, for whom I was very grateful. The 'Care Calendar' designed by Rebecca and Lisa proved to be the most fulfilling. Lisa, who had graduated the year before, announced my plight to her class' social media page while Rebecca, set to graduate in just a few short months, kept her classmates apprised. Thanks to these collective efforts, I found my house becoming a popular destination. Nonetheless, the students who stopped by were very dignified, many of them choosing to drop only off their gift and then make a swift departure. It was readily apparent respecting the student-teacher boundary was essential to all of us.

I have never eaten so well in my life and had to restrain myself from gaining too much weight. One caring student named Katie dropped off delicious stuffed peppers while Sarah dropped off some award-winning lasagna. Felicia dropped off coffee and international fare from our iconic Westside Market. Christie dropped off a pan of her mom's 'Company Chicken,' whose recipe was a closely guarded family secret. On October 10th Tara even dropped off a complete meal from a local restaurant chain, particularly meaningful since it was my mom's birthday. The next day, Christine even brought a most delicious homemade soup with vegetables grown in her garden.

Many students, both current and former, stopped by as their schedules allowed during the day for lunch and good conversation. During their visits, most of the discussion was light banter, and I was touched by their efforts to cheer me up. Steve, however, seized the moment over lunch one day to discuss his transition into the nursing profession. The discussion was very fulfilling and fanned the flames of my desire to return to work.

A former student (and former member of the US armed forces) named Starr came one Saturday morning with her two pre-teen children to mow my lawn. "I'm not taking no for an answer, Dr. Foley. It needs it, and we're already here."

"OK, only if you let me pay them."

"No way. They need to put in community service hours for their school, and this definitely counts. Now, where's the lawnmower?" Starr remained outside with her children while they worked, but I invited them in for snacks and conversation. I encouraged them (including Starr) to focus on their educations and learned of their plans for the future.

How I struggled with these acts of kindness. I had no problem *giving*…a great deal, and very often…but I discovered I had trouble receiving. After much reflection, I decided my internal conflict must be related to nothing more than pride. I thus choose to divest my discomfort in receiving by making a vow to pay back these acts of kindness many times over in the future.

Even with the steady flow of company, love, and support, I still felt useless deep down. I missed my work and comfortable, sedate routine. First thing Monday morning, I called the Plastics Hand Surgeon to ask him when I could return to work, even on a limited-duty or part-time basis. He told me he would see me at my follow-up appointment, which, after all, was only two days away. Until then, I would have to wait. Why was I in such a rush? I could offer no coherent response other than I was bored, and he assured me that was perfectly normal. "Relax and try to enjoy this downtime," he said.

Uh-huh.

In some ways, I felt like a child counting down the days until Christmas and was so happy when it was time for the appointment. The Surgeon looked at my right hand's X-ray and scrutinized my right hand. In keeping with the Orthopedics vs. Plastics Hand distinction, he didn't inquire about nor examine my left arm.

Fine with me, as I suspect my right arm is what's preventing me from returning to work.

He listened intently as I described my daily duties: lecturing, answering emails and phone calls, attending committee meetings, and advising students. Those duties required very little use of my hands, and my mouth was healing quickly enough, except for the significant 'globby' bit of tissue along the incision line inside my mouth.

I often wondered if they were only being kind, but one of the visitors to my home came right out and said, "…it hardly looked like anything had happened to your face. David, whoever did the plastic surgery did a great job!" *Thank you so very much, Senior Plastic Surgery Resident Rachel. You met your end of the bargain by at least not making me any uglier than I was before the accident. Smile…*

"The mass of tissue you are feeling is just scar tissue. Your mouth is still healing, so be careful, but you need to massage the scar tissue gently between your thumb and forefinger. Do that several times a day, and over time, the size of the scar tissue will decrease. Anyway, aren't you concerned about your appearance? I mean getting up in front of the class…."

"No, not at all." I countered. "The students are Nurses in training, and I'm sure they have already seen far worse than this in their clinicals."

"How will you get to work?" he asked.

"I will have a co-worker drive me."

I had an answer prepared for every one of his anticipated questions. Although I hadn't asked, I knew Our Lady of Perpetual Pain Relief would help, as she lived close by and observed a similar work schedule. She had already helped me with my physical pain; now, I hoped she would help me address another type of pain…boredom!

"Do you have help around the house?" the interrogation continued.

"Yes, I have been very blessed in that area."

Keep the questions coming, doctor. I have thought this through.

Long, breathless, and tense silence.

"Ok, I will dictate a return to work letter *with limited duties*. You can pick it up tomorrow afternoon."

"Thank you, Doctor. I really appreciate that." And I sincerely *did* appreciate it.

Ellen took me to pick up the letter the next day, and I was delighted by its contents. My Surgeon had actually listened and took note of my job duties. The letter contained affirmation that I could fulfill all of my responsibilities but suggested I shouldn't drive or lift anything greater than 5 pounds. It was just perfect. I scanned and emailed it to the School's Program Administrator immediately. Predictably, the phone rang about two hours later. I responded to *his* barrage of questions: why was I in such a rush to return to work (*because I'm bored*), was I *ready* to return to work (*yes, please read the letter signed by my Surgeon*), and to provide a general accounting of my health status (*again, please read the letter signed by my Surgeon*).

Another long, breathless silence.

Could he say no? Then what would I do, complain to HR? The Teacher's Union? Please, I don't want to go through all that. Just read the letter…

"OK, you can come back on Monday. That's when your doctor said you could return. Please keep me posted." Quick good-bye then silence.

Just like that. On Monday, I could return to work and rampant—well almost—rampant normalcy. Despite the physical and psychological trauma, I had recovered quickly enough to return to work after only 17 days, known to me as my highly-prized '17 Days in Safety'. Immediately after the accident, I would have thought such swift progress unthinkable, and now here I was, ready to get back in the saddle.

My first day back was blissfully eventful. I got up early and was ready when Our Lady of Perpetual Pain Relief's car pulled into the driveway. I couldn't manage to open the car door, so she had to lean over and open it for me. I also could not wear my usual shirt and tie but decided a more casual appearance was perfectly appropriate given the circumstances. Bill had helped me find an ID holder and key ring to go around my neck, and in it, I placed only my university ID, driver's license, a few dollars, and two keys. Everything I needed would be right there around my neck, and to tell the truth, it felt great to be traveling so light.

I was very nervous entering the School of Nursing, even more than my first day four and a half years earlier. I slipped into my office via a little-used back hallway, but word of my return spread quickly, and several faculty and staff stopped by to offer me their well-wishes—and express their concern about returning to work 'too fast.' I thanked each of them and, when the parade ended, quickly closed my door.

The first order of business was to present a Nursing 100 lecture, and I arrived at the classroom very early to load my lecture onto the sympodium. I always advised my students to arrive at their presentation sites early to work out any technical issues and, more importantly, enhance their confidence by connecting with the presentation space. This advanced preparation served me well, and I delivered my first return-to-work lecture with confidence and without difficulty.

Touchingly, these first-year, first-semester Nursing 100 students were incredibly supportive. They applauded as I entered the room and remained at rapt attention during the whole session. I didn't have to expel any of the usual energy in calling the class to order or quell any side conversations. They even offered to carry items, reminded me not to fall, laughed a little more loudly at my jokes, and slipped greeting cards under my door. Most of all, they bought me a stuffed cat named Oliver, who was dressed in scrubs and sat waiting to greet me on the podium.

Later that day, I presented a Psychiatric-Mental Health lecture to the Junior Class. As part of the course content, I focused on internalizing Erikson's Stages of Psychosocial Development and the concepts of self-efficacy and locus of control. I couldn't resist revisiting, even for a moment, reviewing the Newman Systems Model we had discussed the year before in Nursing 100, and I admit I became teary-eyed when I thanked them all for being part of my 'lines of defense.' The process of retrieving anecdotes from my trauma had begun, and I sensed they would add depth to my teaching practice, starting that very day.

One very nice student named Cody answered a rather complex question, and I absent-mindedly tried to give him a thumbs up. My right thumb wasn't at all cooperative, and the room became quiet. I locked eyes with him and said, "I'll make a deal with you. I'm giving you a virtual thumbs-up *now,* but I will give you the real thing by the end of the semester!" Like many other students,

Cody took my accident in stride and silently conveyed that my standing there with a healing facial deformity, cast, and split was no big deal at all. They all seemed genuinely glad to have me back, and I was very touched.

All in all, I only missed seventeen calendar days, but it seemed so much longer. Thanks to a holiday and pre-scheduled guest speakers, I had missed only a few sessions of each class. In retrospect, I should have taken more time off to rest and heal. I had never missed a day in my four and one-half years at this University and certainly didn't have a reputation for being a slackard. On the other hand, I had been urged by a friend and fellow faculty member to sit out the entire semester and possibly longer, and "....milk this for all it's worth," but I knew I couldn't do that. My values and internal constitution just wouldn't allow it.

To my amazement, however, my decision to return to work so quickly was ultimately viewed with suspicion and perhaps outright disdain by the School of Nursing's Program Administrator. Despite his initial tenuous support for my triumphant return to work, without warning, he decided my return-to-work letter was not descriptive enough and asked for more detailed information. One tense phone call and revised letter from my Surgeon later, he finally seemed satisfied. I guess he was concerned I was overdoing it. Still, my Surgeon countered that although I might need some extra time, it was okay for me to teach classes, answer emails, advise students, attend committee meetings, and all other essential duties associate with my faculty role.

Extra time.

My usual modus operandi was to move quite faster than everyone else, so slowing down just a bit wouldn't make me an outlier but rather push me into the 'normal' part of the faculty bell curve. I was fine with that and hoped the school's Program Administrator would find it at least minimally acceptable.

With Bill in Detroit and my sister back in her regular routine, I basked in my return to rampant, structured, and carefully contrived normalcy. After all, I had now passed '*Twenty* Days in Safety,' and I looked forward to that number growing in abundance. I carefully constructed a nightly routine that would support a stress-free morning: pack my lunch, lay out my clothing, and shower. I could fly through these activities on a typical morning, but these weren't ordinary times.

One ongoing annoyance was my driving restriction. Our Lady of Perpetual Pain Relief continued to pick me up—and drop me off—each day, but the arrangement lasted only two weeks. I just hated to inconvenience her, especially once I learned on some occasions she was kind enough to drop me off in the evening, only to drive back downtown to finish her work. She was also a strong ally in that she encouraged me to proceed with caution, manage expectations and not push the envelope too much those first few weeks. I had respected her as a close friend and co-worker for several years; she would now be memorialized in perpetuity as a saint.

Despite her sage advice, I must admit I was a very non-compliant patient. I started by sneaking in short driving trips to the local supermarket but began driving myself to work shortly after that.

The first time she caught me pulling into the University's parking lot, she laughed but then scolded me. Even though I was sheepish, I wonder how many other middle-aged, fiercely independent people would also grow tired of 'bothering' friends and relatives and wind up overlooking restrictions. Outing myself to the Surgeon at my next follow-up appointment, I told him I was driving and had no choice.

He was very understanding but said the big concern about my driving was the inability to maneuver the steering wheel quickly enough in an emergency. He said he preferred I not drive until both of my arm casts came off in about four more weeks but also recognized he couldn't be there to hold my hand (*please don't*), so the decision to drive or not was up to me.

Hmmmmmmmm

Ok, I saw his point, but I *did* learn an adapted method of holding the steering wheel to facilitate relatively short trips and go back and forth to work. *Couldn't I drive if I was very cautious? Please…I live alone and almost have to.* Albeit polite, I continued to press until he finally threw up his hands and said, "suit yourself," and turned his back to continue charting in the electronic medical record. Filled with optimism over this small perceived victory, I wondered later if he charted the conversation in my chart to mitigate potential liability. Although I continued to drive, my Surgeon's words echoed back to me two weeks later when a car cut me off on the highway, and I had to react very quickly. Both of my arms ached quite a bit for the next few days, but thanks to Our Lady of Perpetual Pain Relief...and Ibuprofen, I was fine. I did not, however, tell any of this to my Surgeon.

Very foolish, Nurse Foley.

On a more sensible note, I threw myself into my Occupational Therapy exercises and proudly displayed my progress at my bi-weekly appointments. I drove myself back and for to the clinic and was quite transparent about that with Donna, who understandably did not endorse my driving either.

She saw me in a large open area where several patients could be seen at once. As a private person, this communal approach to care didn't resonate with me very much, but I did my best to focus on my efforts. I emphasized some of the procedures I performed during my Nursing career (like starting IVs and dressing changes) required a delicate touch and I was becoming concerned my previous level of skill might not return. I also told Donna I was worried that my right thumb still felt somewhat numb, and she did a test to determine its level of sensitivity.

At first, I was impatient and angry with my lack of progress. Donna sensed that, but she continued in her quiet yet firm approach toward meeting my goals. Undaunted, she gave me more activities to perform at home (like separating two types of beans into different piles) that required increased amounts of fine dexterity.

After weeks of hard work, I can still remember the first time I could touch the tip of my thumb to the tip of my middle finger. I was still a long way off from being able to snap my fingers or touch the tip of my thumb to the tip of my pinky, but progress was being made, and I was ecstatic. I even added a second can of tuna to make 'thumb ups' more challenging.

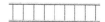

Six weeks later, Bill was back in town and drove me for what I thought was another follow-up appointment with the Plastics Hand Surgeon. Upon arrival to the clinic, a Nurse called for me and said she was going to remove my cast. My cast had served a much-needed purpose to protect my healing arm, but it now smelled sort of like my college roommate, who didn't shower often enough. Yes, it was definitely time to part ways with my malodorous new friend. I assumed I would have a new cast applied for the remainder of my recovery, but as the Nurse turned on the whiny, high-pitched mini-circular saw, she called out, "that's up to your doctor."

Once removed, it *really* smelled. Another Nurse, who never introduced herself, asked me if I would like to keep it as a souvenir. "No," I quickly replied. Thanks for the memories, but just pitch it." She smiled as she tossed the cast in the wastebasket and then instructed me to take the splint off my right wrist and leave it on the exam table. As she walked me down a back corridor, she informed me, "You're going to X-ray. The orders for your films are already in, so just go sign in and then come back to the exam room when you're done."

I felt so naked as I walked without the cast on my left arm and the splint on my right arm, so I kept my arms carefully positioned across my chest during the wait. Marcia was on duty and came from behind the desk to greet me and see how I was progressing. She registered me, took me back for my X-Rays, and soon I navigated back to the exam room in the Plastic Surgery Hand Clinic. My Surgeon arrived breathless and apologetic about a half-hour later, declaring he had been caught up in a traffic jam. I was surprisingly relaxed as he stared intently at my X-rays and carefully examined both arms. He tapped here and there, asking continuously, "Does this hurt?" Each time, I replied "no," wondering if there would be a line at the casting room or if more X-rays would be needed.

"Ok, I'll see you in two months, but only make the appointment if you are having any difficulty. If you have any problems before then, give me a call, and we will get you in right away. In the meantime, *be careful.*" With that, he smiled, turned his back, and began typing on the computer's keyboard in earnest.

Was that it? What was I supposed to do, just…leave?

"Am I getting another cast?" I asked quizzically.

"No, I'll see you in two months."

I sat there in incredulous, amazed silence.

"Do I have to wear the splint?"

"No, let me start over. I'm sorry I am running almost an hour behind, and I guess I'm in too much of a hurry. Your X-rays show adequate healing of the avulsion fracture of your left elbow and left Triquetral fracture, and the surgical repair to your right arm is progressing very well. You don't need another cast, and you should only wear your splint as needed for comfort. Go to your Occupational Therapy appointments and keep working hard. You are recovering well. Just be very careful, and I'll see you in two months, but only if you need to come in. You're done." He put out his large, muscular hand and gently shook mine.

Now, doctor, that's what I call putting therapeutic closure on a provider-patient relationship.

Stunned and overcome with emotion, I started to tear up a bit, and the moment was incredibly awkward for both of us.

"Thank you, doctor." I'll see you later.

I stood up, walked out the exam door, and have not seen him since.

When I entered the waiting room, Bill noticed the expression on my face and looked concerned. As I walked closer toward him, his gaze shifted to my naked arms, and he seemed surprised but also assumed we would now move to the Orthopedics Clinic for another round of casting.

"Nope, I replied, No cast. It's over. I will come back in two months, but only if I have any problems." As we walked to the car, I told him what happened in more detail; we sat in silence for a few moments and then left. Free from my cast and splint, I celebrated the small victory of opening the car door without assistance. With the cast removed, my left arm felt light and movement effortless.

It seemed a celebration was in order, so we stopped for breakfast and then drove right to a beautiful park to admire the fall leaves amid the splendor of a beautiful Midwestern fall afternoon. Marveling at God's creation seemed the perfect way to celebrate the loss of my cast, split, and post-op visits.

I still had Occupational Therapy appointments ahead, but I looked forward to them. I knew insurance only paid for a certain number of visits, so I decided to make as much progress as possible in the shortest amount of time. I performed my exercises at home, during red lights, in my office, waiting in line at the grocery store… anywhere I had a free moment. On more than one occasion, someone observed me doing 'squeezes' and other hand exercises, eliciting curious stares, but who cared? I had moved into another phase of recovery, and that's all that mattered.

The day was complete when I called my parents, and I announced we were going out to dinner. I told them I just *had* to get out of the house and experience more of the beautiful unseasonably warm fall weather. I never really enjoyed eating al fresco, but another nearby park's dining pavilions had just been renovated, and I suggested we dine there. We put together a simple picnic, and when I took off my jacket to surprise them with my bare arms, the picnic quickly turned into a celebration. It felt so fulfilling to actually pour their beverage or hand them their meal, albeit clumsily. The warmth and laughter which followed confirmed the venue was the right choice for this celebratory dinner.

We heard the weather report had called for a drastic change in the weather within a few hours. One reporter said something like, "This is going to be the last warm evening for a while, so if you're going to do something outside, do it tonight!" Well, we did, and it was the perfect evening. The dramatic change in the weather happened within an hour after we arrived home and seemed to symbolize one season ending and another beginning. We even woke up to a dusting of snow the following day, and somehow everything seemed so right.

Goodbye fall, 2016, with all your pain and challenges.

Hello, winter 2016-17! I certainly hope you bring the familiarity and routine I have been missing of late.

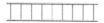

With the support of my family, friends, faculty, and staff, I was able to get through the remainder of the semester with dignity. Thanksgiving, in particular, was joyful in so many ways. With nearly '60 Days in Safety', it was a day for gratitude and to acknowledge the semester was nearly over. When the last final grade was posted a few weeks later, I left for Christmas break with mixed feelings. I was so thankful to be alive, yet realized I had so much to accomplish to get back on track with my ambitious post-doctoral agenda.

Throughout the holiday season, I realized how lucky I was that no one responded affirmatively to the attending's question, "did he hit his head?" I was so fortunate to have the ability to hear the question, cognitively process it, and be the first to respond a resounding "no!" Offensive to the Physician or not, it was my voice, the voice of his patient, to offer the opinion I had not suffered a head trauma; otherwise, the story might have had a much different ending. A relative later shared one of their co-workers fell from a ladder and hit his head on the concrete, resulting in a closed head injury, an extended stay in Neuro Rehab, and ultimately, early retirement due to permanent cognitive limitations.

Well aware of what might have been, I tapped into a growing sense of peace during Christmas break and worked to catch up with a sense of quiet purpose. In deference to the Surgeon's warning to "be careful," I limited my work to two hours per day and even at that typed gingerly with my arms comfortably resting on pillows. I decided that even without an injury, two hours was long enough to work over the holidays anyway. I needed the time to renew and restore, especially now.

I finalized the draft of an article, submitted it for publication, and completed other work that had been languishing on my computer's desktop. Always one to plan in advance, some of the work had a January 1st deadline, so I was glad I had made good progress before the accident in September.

Careful planning, a foundational element of my life's narrative.

Days in safety thankfully continued to grow, and grow, and grow in number.

PART VIII

ONWARD IN SAFETY

CHAPTER 18

MORE THAN 1000 DAYS IN SAFETY

Nothing is impossible. The word itself says 'I'm possible.'
Audrey Hepburn

T HE CALENDAR TELLS me it has been greater than three years since the accident, which means I have lived over 1000 Days in Safety. The time off immediately following the accident gave me so much time to reflect on my life, and I ultimately concluded that my work had *been my life* for so many years. 'Work to live, don't live to work' was an expression I heard on TV, and I adopted it as a new personal philosophy. I thought so much about what I did for a living. Professors must publish, research and teach, but it is teaching that truly captivates me and thus falls into the 'work to live' category. Though necessary, the rest now feels a bit secondary.

Despite my injuries, I acknowledge that my profession as a Nurse educator affords me the rare and highly gratifying opportunity to witness my students bring to life the concepts learned in the classroom, skills lab, and clinical settings. Albeit during difficult circumstances involving my care, I had the rare chance to see them use such knowledge, skills, and concepts firsthand. What Nurse educator wouldn't delight in seeing that? With each therapeutic interaction, demonstration of skill, or attempt to educate, I was the recipient of their amazingly empathic yet safe and technically proficient care. On hundreds of occasions in the past, I had observed them in action, discussed their care, *graded* their care, but it was within the context of them providing care to patients in the student role. This time I was the recipient, and it was so meaningful and fulfilling.

I never fully understood which of them were assigned as my Nurse or if they stopped by just to see me. Nonetheless, I will never forget their acts of caring as they practiced the art and science of nursing. I also realized they needed me to let go and allow them to be the Nurse in the equation. Those who stopped in only to say hello perhaps simply wanted me to see them in their new role: *"I'm in uniform; I passed the NCLEX-RN! I may have struggled through school, but here I am—I made it!"* Many were the first in their families to graduate from college, while others had to work full-time to pay their tuition and support themselves. I would be very proud and want one of my former instructors to see me in action, too, albeit under better circumstances.

The power equation had certainly changed in that room. I was no longer a teacher but their patient. I was the 'mannequin,' and my voice, eyes, facial grimacing, and body language were all saying, "help me…and no, this is not a classroom exercise!" It was admittedly quite odd that I was very reluctant to allow them to see my vulnerability and deflected by referencing concepts we learned in class. It was an obvious ploy that got me through those awkward moments, but I am sure they figured that out on their own.

Months after my discharge, I heard a former student—and one of my caregivers during my hospital stay—address the current student body as a Nursing Student Alumni Association representative. In reference to changes in lifestyle required to meet the demands of the nursing program, he said, "do you know what an externalized locus of control is? Be sure to ask Dr. Foley, and he will explain it to you." After the nervous laughter subsided, he shared his thoughts on losing control and independence based on the demands of the nursing program. "Get ready for the biggest challenge of your life," he told them, but when he glanced over at me, we shared a silent moment that spoke volumes. I knew the next time I covered the concept of locus of control in class, I would speak from my own very personal place, one that I hoped would help produce even more empathic Nurses.

I was tempted to contact the attending Physician from Trauma Bay 1 and thank him for his care. I wondered if he would remember me, but then again, I suspect I might be a patient he has not soon forgotten. I hope he and I can speak at length someday and even co-facilitate a lecture to an inter-disciplinary audience on the importance of therapeutic communication. I know that might sound strange to some, but it seems like a very sensible and intriguing opportunity as an educator. I gained much insight into my own psycho-social needs, nursing skills, and teaching practice on the day I experienced my literal 'post doc crash.' I wistfully hoped we could collaborate to present the experience of our time together in Trauma Bay 1 to an interdisciplinary audience of students and seasoned hospital staff.

That hasn't happened yet, but I have accepted every opportunity to speak, teach, and consult, all in hopes of enhancing safe patient care. I find my work coming from a very private space, especially since the accident shifted my perspective and taught me how much my mission—and people—mean to me. In the two years following, I made every effort possible to return to rampant normalcy, but as is often the case, those efforts were thwarted by the waves of change resulting from such a significant event. If nothing else, the accident proved I could adapt quickly based on a strong sense of personal resilience and self-efficacy. My 'lines of defense' were challenged, but in the end, they were strengthened. My relationships with the people who rallied around me are more profound than ever, and my self-concept is more hardy as a result.

Despite these successes, however, my life is now bounded by a certain sense of pragmatism tempered with just a dash of cynicism. Sitting on the garage floor in unbelievable pain with blood flowing down my face on that beautiful September afternoon, I sensed the first whispers of my mortality, and I no longer view myself as untouchable. I am vulnerable to the same risks as everyone else, and yes, bad things can—and do—happen in my world. It might have once seemed exhilarating to speed recklessly to my nursing school clinicals; after all, I certainly didn't want to be late, did I? Looking back, I am surprised an accident didn't find me much sooner. When it did on that September afternoon in 2016, I could never imagine returning to a space where I could view life, even peripherally, through the brash, unfiltered lens of young adulthood. No, I had passed a point of no return and grown up. Though I certainly couldn't have known it in those few terrible moments following the fall, I would emerge several months later a stronger person emotionally, psychologically, and spiritually and for that, I give thanks.

My most significant frustration was, and continues to be, some subtle physical limitations. Although my right hand has almost been restored to its pre-accident state, I now drop at least four objects per day. In fact, it has become a joke in my circle of family and friends. I seem to have difficulty sensing how strongly I am grasping an object and must be very mindful of anything in my hand. Although I remain in practice as a PRN Nurse, I am glad my practice setting in Psychiatric-Mental Health doesn't require procedures that require fine motor skills like starting intravenous lines. Instead, I use my mind and voice to engage patients with therapeutic communication and perform psychosocial assessments. I always feel so enthusiastic when I am in practice, not only because I love working with patients but also because I walk in gratitude that I can still do it. I sincerely hope that gratitude is evident to the patients I serve. I wish I could share more with them about my own experiences, but appropriate self-disclosure is always in order.

Despite my optimism and the opportunities for self-discovery provided by this experience, I still search for more. During my accident and initial recovery, I made a concerted effort to lean heavily into the role of the patient, exploring its every boundary and making as many connections as I possibly could between theoretical knowledge, life experience, and clinical practice. I reflected that nursing education falls rather neatly into three settings: the classroom, nursing resource lab, and clinicals. Since I have taught in all three settings, I brought experiences from all three into the role of patient, even as I sat in my garage moments after the accident. I knew my life had changed, but remained uncertain of the outcome. As my care progressed, I did my best not to be critical but simply remain observant.

As a clinical instructor, I often point out examples of poor vs. exemplary nursing practice to students. The chance to interact with the Trauma Team was humbling and quite frankly terrifying, but the short trip on a gurney up a few floors to the inpatient Trauma Unit was transformative. I was delighted—and surprised—to be greeted by former students whose budding nursing practices were partially shaped by *me*. Dressed in their respective uniforms, they gathered around me to say, 'how can we help you?' I sensed, however, it was also to say 'thank you.' Such was the essence of these encounters—my pride of being an educator intersecting with their pride at being in practice. That pride was a curious source of empowerment, even as my locus of control was not only externalized, but seemed miles away.

Thanks in part to the care I received from my valued, though disjointed, interdisciplinary team, the terror long-term disability slowly turned to the joy of recovery, but not in that inpatient unit. Despite the personal connections with my students, I couldn't wait to leave. Feelings of safety and security didn't start to emerge until I returned home, a space of protection defined by physical, emotional, and spiritual factors.

Within the safety of my home front, I had much time to think and realized my life was far off course. I resolved to capture the essence of the little boy who ran to greet his father every evening at the entrance to the kitchen door, anxious to hear about the happenings of someone else's day and concerned only about that moment in time. That little guy was bursting with enthusiasm and was firmly grounded in the joy of his being with no worries about tomorrow. He was happy and satisfied with so very little. Separating him and me were many years of life experiences, including school, college, hospital administration, and nursing. I had no idea if reconnecting with my little self was even possible, but I resolved to try.

A one-second trip straight down from a ladder's summit to a concrete floor created an opportunity to rediscover *me,* and now I must do it. Amazingly, I left the University where I both worked and earned my doctoral degree, somehow realizing a new vision for my future was the best way to reconnect with the past. Despite the wonderful support of students and colleagues, I firmly believe the Program Administrator's initial lack of support was what pointed me toward the door.

The doctoral program was transformative as I embraced learning opportunities, yet I felt my sense of scholarly inquiry had become stagnant in the year following the accident. The way forward was to spend time with people who knew far more than I did, hence my decision to join the nursing faculty of another nearby school with a solid reputation for scholarly inquiry. Being around brilliant, accomplished educators and researchers who have created nursing leaders and innovators at the local, national, and international levels rekindled in me an adult version of my child-like enthusiasm.

At least one evening each week, I have my mom and dad over for dinner at my house, and I share many exciting stories with them. I don't always agree with the opinions of my new colleagues. Still, it is a pleasure to take home interesting stories to share with the people who gave me life and raised me within a beautiful and enduring narrative of safety.

I remain concerned about some physical limitations, especially my right hand and upper arm, but keep performing the exercises recommended by the physical therapist in hopes of a full recovery. Second only to my abounding faith in God and love for my family, teaching continues to be my life's work and is the reason I move forward loving, living, and nursing...in safety and gratitude.

EPILOGUE: 2021 AND ONWARD

They are the things that fill our lives with comfort and our hearts with gladness -- just the pure air to breathe and the strength to breath it; just warmth and shelter and home folks; just plain food that gives us strength; the bright sunshine on a cold day; and a cool breeze when the day is warm.
Laura Ingalls Wilder

TO DATE, I have now lived in over 1500 'Days of Safety.' I can only imagine how ecstatic my dad's Safety Team would be in boasting such a record. Although the experience was terrifying and life-altering, I latched onto the goal I set in the Emergency Room's lobby and have shared many rich experiences with my students through anecdotes, simulations, and case studies. Unfortunately, my suitcase of stories is now so large and unwieldy I am no longer able to carry it with me. However, through practice, I have learned to leave it safely in storage and retrieve it only when necessary. In doing so, I feel less burdened and free to move forward.

Despite much hard work, I *still* have some residual numbness in my right thumb and try not to become frustrated when I continue to drop my quota of at least four objects per day. On good days, the object might be a pen, but it is a cup of coffee or an essential document on others. Those incidents aren't amusing, but recalling the many hours I spent wondering if I would regain use of my hand at all, my imperfection reminds me just how far I have come.

I continue in part-time nursing practice and, in doing so, lean deeply into the art of nursing. For years I told students nursing is an art and a science, but I now feel it in my whole being. Practicing therapeutic communication and mindfulness in pursuit of an effective Nurse-Patient relationship takes finesse, insight, and cultural competence as well as technical skill. In my opinion, the shimmering complexities of the art of nursing make my profession transcend the realities of science.

I often sit with patients and take just a moment to ground myself before speaking. When I look into their eyes, I see pain, hope, anxiety, depression, and various other emotions. As others have so generously done for me, I recognize the importance of seeing them from a holistic perspective, recognizing their strengths and challenges.

More often than not, I leave a shift feeling more enriched than before. I don't want to be one of those psychiatric Nurses who take permanent residence behind the relative safety of the glassed-in Nurses station, but rather one who embraces opportunities to engage patients as often as I can. Family, friends, and students took so many opportunities to engage in many acts of caring for me; I now view my nursing practice as the chance to pay the goodness and caring forward.

Settling the score again, only this time the right way.

I proceed more deliberately and carefully through life, constantly recalling my onomatopoeic trip on the ladder one beautiful afternoon. Enmeshed in the 'if only I had' syndrome, I approach situations, ranging from everyday routines to novel experiences, from the perspective of safety and do my best to instill caution in my students. I wonder if I have become my father. *Probably not*, I tell myself, but perhaps just a bit more than before. The word safety has more meaning now than ever, and discussions about safe, patient-centered care continue to be commonplace. I no longer ask students to simply recall safety principles but apply them through case studies, simulations, reflections, and meaningful discussions. The QSEN (Quality, Safety, and Education for Nurses) Principles, for example, have become an integral part of my teaching—and life—practices. Engaging students in the classroom and clinical settings with opportunities to improve patient care through rapid-cycle performance improvement has proven very fruitful. "Anyone can recite the QSEN

Principles," I tell them, "but can you actually *apply* them to real-life situations."

I attempt to guide them through the process of examining teamwork and collaboration, safety, and patient-centered care from a very personal perspective. Time spent in the Trauma Bay, Trauma Unit, Surgical Suite, and Outpatient Occupational Therapy were a series of highly instructive and introspective scenarios in real-life application. My decision at the threshold of the Emergency Department to transcend pain by navigating into a space of personal and intellectual discovery is something for which I can honestly give thanks. What if I had just closed my eyes and disappeared into the abyss that beckoned me? I would have missed the silent but meaningful glances of those in the waiting room as Erica pushed me with such purpose. In fact, I would have missed out on meeting Erica altogether, albeit briefly. I would have also lost the opportunity to observe the fascinating interpersonal dynamics in Trauma Bay 1 and, worse yet, might have mistakenly given the impression that I was far less alert and oriented than I was. I pushed through the pain and am so grateful I was able to do that. Five years on, I believe I am a better Nurse and Nurse educator thanks to those experiences.

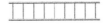

I recall my initial impressions about my world where nothing bad ever happened. The safety of that world provided me with a childhood bounded only by the expanses of my imagination. Oh, to be live in such an unconstrained space today. I can, however, create a similar enviornment of unbridled, thoughtful inquisitiveness for my students; the classroom as an incubator—a warm, nurturing environment where bad things *can* happen, but only for a brief moment. I leverage the potential of transporting my students to places where bad things do happen through the use of simulation or carefully constructed situations that mimic 'low incidence, high-risk scenarios. They are 'low-incidence' because they occur very infrequently and thus would hopefully never be encountered by my students in the clinical setting. They are also 'high-risk' because they involve Patient-Patient or Patient-Nurse, or Nurse-Nurse interactions that are often extremely dangerous.

Energized by the opportunity to expose students to engaging, clinically relevant situations through simulation, I authored many scripts and partnered with acting students to bring them to life in the most realistic manner possible. So many of the characters, albeit in composite form, were taken from my personal experiences as a patient. Mr. Silver-haired 'flunked his skill check' is there, as is Nurse Vivian and her outstanding patient advocacy skills. Even Trauma Bay 1's bespectacled Physician has been immortalized so students can see the benefits of a Medical Model of Care in life-threatening situations.

I encourage my students to throw themselves into the simulations with reckless abandon. Reality, along with the heavy burden of professional responsibility, will come soon enough. For the moment, however, students rest easy that any stress involved with immersion in simulated learning experiences will usually dissipate during the walk from the classroom to the conference room for constructive instructor/peer feedback and debriefing.

It seemed the Nurse educators who instructed me weren't focused much on innovation but rather on structure, order, and discipline. Perhaps that was a result of the nursing culture in which they were educated. I realize now that some of the instructors were nearing retirement age in the late 1990s, meaning some graduated from nursing school and were launched into the highly patriarchal culture of 1950's hospitals. For them, teaching us how to be disciplined Nurses who could successfully navigate a rigid social stratum and thus work to maintain an orderly hospital culture was their job. Concepts like simulation, reflective thinking, and diversity in nursing weren't on the horizon quite yet. After much reflection, I believe the discipline and structure in my administrative and nursing practices directly resulted from how my nursing instructors enculturated me into the profession. That realization has allowed me to place so many of my nursing school experiences in proper context and, in turn, led me to a place of peaceful resolution.

As a proud member of Generation X, I was raised in a world without a military draft or widespread world conflict. Various members of previous generations accordingly labeled us as being soft, undisciplined, and unprepared for adversity. On the other hand, my generation is described as pragmatic, in favor of order and routine, and doesn't require continuous praise and reinforcement. We were often called the 'Baby Bust,' the inglorious aftermath of the world-famous Baby Boomers. As Baby Bust implied, our entrée into society felt just a bit deflated. Nevertheless, I feel proud of our collective description of resilience and fierce independence.

From the podium's bird's eye view, this Generation Xer often wonders what the next generation's epitaph will be. An integral part of my mission has been to coax them out of their safe bubble of social policies and guide them into the world of nursing, where they will witness many things that aren't perfectly safe yet very necessary to nursing practice. On the other hand, I feel extraordinarily encouraged by their collective warmth, openness, tolerance, and generosity, and I don't want to expose them to too much too soon. They might experience their own wake-up call at some point in their lives, but I can only wish love, comfort, and 'Thousands of Days in Safety' to each one of them. I hope not a single student has an experience like a loud, cacophonous metallic ladder hitting a concrete floor, but I know there are no guarantees. For now, I can only present reality from carefully constructed experiences offered by the classroom or nursing skills lab.

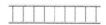

The ultimate test of my recovery came in the spring of 2021. I ascended the same ladder in the very same spot in my garage, but this time I worked as a team with a friend. He held the ladder and made sure it was secure at all times. Rather than avoid it, I embraced the experience, realizing I needed to conquer my fear to truly move forward. Yes, bad things do happen in my world, but I am surrounded by my Faith, love, comfort, knowledge, and because of that, I can move on. I ascended the ladder only to touch the ceiling and then asked my nephew, a gifted craftsman, to hang the brackets for me.

During the past five years, I have accomplished much of what I hoped for lying in bed in the inpatient Trauma Unit. I have published, acted as a co-principal investigator on a large federally-funded grant, gave a commencement address and other guest lectures, served on a national nursing organization's board, and of course, educated many more students.

Although I desperately want to say I have fully recovered, that is simply not the case. Some deficits were undetected during my initial hospitalization, especially since my broken bones and facial laceration demanded all the attention. I have frequent pain in both shoulders, knees, and ankles and wish they had also been assessed at the time of the injury, as perhaps they too might have benefitted from some physical therapy. Nevertheless, a spirit of gratitude takes over, and I am reminded of how quickly I could return to work and resume normal activities. However, with so much success at hand, my accident seems to be the gift that just keeps on giving.

Another unexpected and insidious visitor erodes at my optimism—the specter of depression and its companions of anhedonia, anergia, and avolution. Several months after the accident, it became apparent to everyone that I had recovered physically and resumed all former responsibilities, including my least favorite duty: yard work. I made quite a point, however, of making sure everyone knew I was 'back to normal' and, in essence, told the world, "See, I've fully recovered."

The male ego in action.

As time moved on, I noticed I just couldn't quite get back into my pre-accident routine. I used to love to walk every evening around the neighborhood or, better yet, driving to a local park to take in the beauty of God's creation. I recall going directly to that park on the way home from the 'surprise' removal of both arm casts. It seemed such a logical and familiar stepping stone on the return to normalcy. On days off, I began to notice I just quite couldn't get myself to get out of the recliner and do anything, let alone go for my usual walk.

With the benefit of my Faith, family, friends, and a gifted counselor, I have persevered and continued in my recovery. Each time I share my with others recovering from serious accidents, I feel a bit stronger. Each time I present a topic to an interdisciplinary audience, I feel enriched. Each time I stand before a classroom of students, I draw on their collective strengths. With each of these activities, I move on to a new narrative, and for that, I feel extraordinarily grateful.

Onward and onward....in safety.

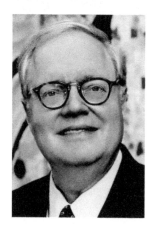

ABOUT THE AUTHOR

Dr. David Foley is a Nurse, Educator, and Administrator who has worked within the complex and often hyper-turbulent northeast Ohio healthcare system for the past 30 years. A Cleveland, Ohio native, he is a proud graduate of a local inner-ring suburban school system and often nostalgically reflects on his well-engrained 1970s-esque narrative of personal safety. A long-time advocate for Nurses, he entered nursing school at the age of 31, intending to meld his administrative and budding clinical experiences to create a unique skill set that eventually settled into a deep desire to educate others. He specifically devoted his doctoral research to exploring factors impacting nursing students who are men, of color, or those with limited English proficiency. In doing so, he brought to peaceful resolution the subtle—and often overt—misandry he experienced in his pre-licensure nursing program. An avid historian and writer, he is highly devoted to his family, both human and feline. His greatest passion, however, remains to teach and serve others.

Made in the USA
Monee, IL
03 September 2021